GET UP!

WHY YOUR CHAIR IS KILLING YOU
AND WHAT YOU CAN DO ABOUT IT

JAMES A. LEVINE, MD, PHD

MAYO CLINIC AND ARIZONA STATE UNIVERSITY

St. Martin's Griffin

New York

www.stmartins.com

Designed by Letra Libre, Inc.

NEAT™ and NEAT® are trademarks and service marks of Mayo Foundation for Medical Education and Research.

The author's affiliation with Mayo Clinic does not constitute an endorsement by Mayo Clinic of the content of this book, or any views or opinions expressed in this book.

Mayo Clinic owns equity in Muve Technologies, Inc. Mayo Clinc and James Levine, MD, PhD, may receive royalties from the sale of products developed and sold by Muve Technologies, Lumo BodyTech Inc and Kersh Health Inc.

Library of Congress Cataloging-in-Publication Data

Levine, James A.
    Get up! : why your chair is killing you and what you can do about it / James A. Levine.
        pages   cm
    Includes index.
    ISBN 978-1-137-27899-9
    1. Exercise. 2. Self-care, Health. 3. Lifestyles. I. Title.
    QP301.L625   2014
    613.7'1—dc23

                                                                    2014000413

Our books may be purchased in bulk for promotional, educational, or business use. Please contact your local bookseller or the Macmillan Corporate and Premium Sales Department at (800) 221-7945, extension 5442, or by e-mail at MacmillanSpecialMarkets@macmillan.com.

First published by Palgrave Macmillan, a division of St. Martin's Press LLC

First St. Martin's Griffin Edition: July 2014

D   10   9   8   7

For my lab:

Shelly, Gabe, Chinmay and Samantha

CONTENTS

INTRODUCTION

HOW CAN MY CHAIR BE KILLING ME?

Can chairs kill us?[1] We sit in them, work in them, shop in them, eat in them and date in them. We live amid a sea of chairs. In this book I argue that chairs—adjustable, swivel, recliner, sofa, couch, four-legged, three-legged, wooden, plastic, dining and bar—all of them—are out to get us, to harm us, to kill us.

Chair addiction—like the alcoholic thirsting for another Scotch—is the constant need we have developed to sit. We slouch from bed to car seat, to work seat, to sofa. The cost is too great; for every hour we sit, two hours of our lives walk away—lost forever. The list of health consequences is an alphabet soup of life's torments. A is for arthritis, B is for blood pressure, C is for cancer, D is for diabetes . . . and so it goes. But what I have learned is that it is *not* these health consequences that hurt people the most. Sedentary living etches away at our very essence. The spring in our step has vanished. We sit in our cubicles alone, blue and sad. Our chairs have become islands of isolation.

My colleagues and I have developed and delivered chair-release schemes to more than 60 corporations and dozens of schools. Walking through cube land in a contemporary corporation is rather like ambling around a morgue. The malaise of the modern American workplace is a contemporary cry of misery: "Free us!" Chair-sentenced workers would cry out and rise up—if only they had time enough away from their screens to do so. The sitting disease is about far more than the health consequences ABCs—the sitting disease is about sentencing the modern soul to sedentariness. Together we are all dying a slow death—body, mind and soul—glued to our chairs.

BUT WE SIT EVERY DAY. PEOPLE HAVE SAT FOR CENTURIES. HOW CAN SITTING BE HARMFUL?

How can something that we do so many times each day hurt us? It seems implausible. But there are other things we do many times each day that have become unhealthy. Take eating: We eat several times every day. But do you need convincing as to how harmful eating has become? Eating, like sitting, is life threatening when done to excess and in the wrong way. Tens of thousands of studies have shown that *nutricide* (killing oneself with food) comes from overdosing our body with foods that most often resemble products from a chemistry experiment than natural foodstuffs. Yet we have to eat. Eating is essential for life—when undertaken in the right frequency, with the correct ingredients and at the appropriate dose. The same can be said for sitting.

The goal of sitting is to give our bodies a break from standing, which is the way the human anatomy and physiology is designed. Human design is to be upright for most of the day: walking at work, walking and nurturing our young, walking while inventing, walking while gathering our food, running on the hunt. Sitting, we know from studies in rural populations,[2] is supposed to be undertaken in short batches to break up the motion of a dynamic day. But the opposite has become the modern way; we sit for 13 hours a day, sleep for 8 and move for 3. Living all day on our bottoms wrecks our health.

I have spent the last 25 years running the anti-chair movement from my laboratory at Mayo Clinic in Rochester, Minnesota. In our nonexercise activity thermogenesis (NEAT) laboratory, my colleagues and I develop counter-chair maneuvers, and we investigate the harm sitting does to both body and mind.

In the pages that follow, we delve into history to understand how the chair sentence came into existence without us apparently noticing; after all, sitting hurts more people's health than smoking. We head to agricultural communities—sit-free zones—and chart the impact of modernity. We examine the history of the chair in order to better understand our enemy so that we are better armed to conquer the chair and its overlord, The Chairman. We walk into the lab to understand not only why sitting is harmful but also what happens to our brains as a consequence of the chair sentence. We then amble through an art studio to see what modern sedentariness is doing to our vanishing creative flair and switch on the TV to see how artistry reflects society—Homer Simpson, the modern man (*Homo sedentarius*).

But this is not a book of doom and gloom. I discuss a series of solutions that range from self-reinvention to environmental redesign. Your first step is to take the chair test to see whether you are a victim of The Chairman: whether you are a chair captive.

THE CHAIR TEST

As with eating, there are healthy chair habits. But just as nutricide kills, so too does chair addiction. To learn whether you are a chair addict, complete this simple test. Answer yes or no to each question.

1. Do you work seated on a chair?
2. Have you ever shopped on the Internet?
3. Do you watch TV sitting for one hour a day or more?
4. Do you ever eat while watching TV or in the car?
5. Have you ever Internet dated?
6. Do you own a recliner?
7. If you go to a party, do you seek out a chair?
8. Look at your sofa. Does it have an imprint of your buttocks?
9. Do you spend more time with friends electronically than in real life?

10. Have you ever fantasized about or engaged in sexual intercourse while in a chair?

SCORING

Give yourself 1 point for each yes answer.

0:	Close the book and give it to a friend.
1–2:	Chair pre-addict
3–5:	Chair addict
6–8:	Chair imprisoned
9–10:	Chairaholic

LET'S MOVE ON

When you first contemplate a book about the harm of sitting, you may view it as absurd. How can chairs possibly kill anyone? Perhaps you expect a book sugarcoated in magazine-style triviality like the quiz you just completed. However, this book summarizes 40 years of science—the work of scores of scientists and physicians from around the world. The scientific conclusion is clear: Humans are not designed to sit all day long, from a physiological, medical, creative or psychological perspective. Sitting is like a terrible diet; it has crept up on us as a consequence of modernity. The evidence is in. If, by the end of this book, you are not convinced by the arguments and the data, I have failed you. But, please, I beg of you, read with an open mind. Scientific bodies such as the National Institutes of Health, public health organizations and even governments recognize that your chair is shaving years off your life and the lives of everyone who sits around you. If you scored *any* points on The Chair Test, you are probably at risk. Cut the chains, get up from your chair, unlock your mind and read on.

PART I

THE CHAIRMAN'S RISE TO POWER

1

IN THE BEGINNING

A WANDERING POND SNAIL

A piece of chalk flies from the hand of the schoolmaster and misses the boy asleep at the back of class 5M by a good six inches. The rest of the boys chuckle. The boy asleep is a chubby 11-year-old with dark hair. He is in the M stream, the bottom tier at Colet Court School in London. M does not stand for moron, as the other boys in the school would have it; it stands for mediocre. The teacher is Mr. Lewison, six foot two inches tall, young, with long shoulder-length brown hair; he was once a top graduate from Cambridge University. Again, he takes aim and fires another piece of chalk at the boy. Mr. Lewison's double major was in English and psychology, not chalk throwing. The second piece of chalk misses the boy's left ear. The rest of the class laughs. The third piece hits the center of the boy's forehead; I wake up. "Levine, welcome back to *Julius Caesar*," Mr. Lewison calls across the room. "Come and see me at the end of class." If ever there was a chair comfortable enough to sit in and a lesson boring enough to fall asleep in, Mr. Lewison's 5M English class was it. But it was not Mr. Lewison's fault entirely that I repeatedly fell asleep; I had not had an uninterrupted night's sleep for months. I didn't sleep a whole night through because I was infatuated by Joanne.

JOANNE—MY FIRST TRUE LOVE

I cannot explain quite how I became infatuated with Joanne at the age of 11. It is a natural age for a boy to feel yearnings of the heart since by then hormones have begun their campaign. But it was not girls that dominated my nights and dreams. My heart had been stolen by Joanne Lymnaeidae—a pond snail.

Love is a strange mistress, and I must confess that I was not monogamous; two snails possessed my devotion, Joanne and Maurice, both acquired from the lake in Regents Park. Worse still, there were other snails before Maurice and Joanne, but we will not discuss their fates. Suffice it to say, snail-rearing is an art form that takes several snails to master. (If snail love strikes you too, one trick of the trade I will share is that cats view pond snails that live under your bed as a delicacy.)

What's an 11-year-old boy doing with snails? Over several weeks I had spent my allowance on building a large, thin fish tank. It was about three feet long, two feet tall, but only four inches wide. I had bought each piece of glass from a local glazier and joined them together with silicone glue. The tank constantly leaked water, but not badly. Each night at just before 9 p.m. (bedtime) I would remove either Joanne or Maurice from bowls under my bed and attach her/him (they are hermaphroditic) to the inside of the tank. Once the snail attached, I would mark the spot with a thick red marker on the outside of the glass. Then I set my alarm clock for an hour later, for 10 p.m. At 10 p.m., I woke up and marked where the snail had moved to, and then I set my alarm for 11 p.m. and went back to sleep. I woke up at 11 p.m., marked the snail's progress and reset the alarm for midnight. I did this every hour through the night until 7 a.m. At 7 a.m. I traced the red markings onto parchment paper, dated the paper and replaced the snail under my bed. I did this every night for two years, working with many new loves: many other snails.

CONFRONTATION

I told Mr. Lewison about my snail-tracking project. "What on earth are you doing this for?" Mr. Lewison asked me after class. I explained that I had a theory that each snail advanced with a fixed pattern of movement unique to it. I believed that each snail was wired to move in a certain way—that every snail has a certain predefined style of motion. I hypothesized that Joanne would always move in swirls, whereas Maurice would always slime along in straight lines.

"And do they?" the chalk-flinging master asked.

At that point, I was only a few months in to my experiments, so I told him I did not know.

Mr. Lewison was a young, dynamic teacher who wanted to be viewed as cool by the students, before being cool was cool. "You need to focus on your schoolwork," he told me, but he did not tell me to stop my experiments. I knew that I baffled Mr. Lewison. He had overseen the IQ testing of the entire school year. My score was the highest by 20 points, but I was in the M stream, and I seemed to him as dim as a piece of chalk. He could not figure me out; I kept falling asleep in his English class, and he kept throwing chalk at me. I was consistently second from the bottom. He never asked me about the snails again.

19 SNAILS LATER

I finished my experiments two years later, and, at the age of 13, I was interviewed to enter one of London's most famous schools, St. Paul's. St. Paul's is a classic old British school. It had spawned colonels, senior civil servants and leaders. I showed up with 217 three-foot pieces of parchment paper—each was the overnight pattern of movement from a single snail. The principal of the school, Mr. Hyde, was a thin, wiry man in a dark suit. He looked as if he should be unpleasant (St. Paul's, at that time, used the cane for discipline), but he was not. Mr. Hyde was genuinely interested in the education of his students; he just beat bad behavior out of them. I remember the noise of the pieces of parchment paper shaking in my sweaty hand as I explained my experiments to Mr. Hyde.

"Were you right about your theory?" he asked me.

By then I knew the answer. I explained to him that I was sort of right and kind of wrong. I had originally thought that every snail would move with its own swirl and at a constant distance every night. In that regard I had been wrong. But I was right in another way—each snail had a distinct *style* of movement. Joanne, for instance, always moved in a jagged way—in the pattern of saw teeth—while Maurice consistently moved across the glass smoothly as if following the curve of a shooting star.

Mr. Hyde asked me why I thought that was, and I explained, like a typical scientist, that I would need to undertake further research. My initial bedroom studies trying to dissect pieces of snail brain had not been successful (cat food). I did not tell him this, but I guessed the style of snail movement was hardwired in their brains. No doubt bemused by the snail boy with a surprisingly high IQ, Mr. Hyde admitted me to St. Paul's, and a year later I was awarded the St. Paul's Smee Prize in Science—the youngest boy ever to get it.

I never explained to Mr. Hyde or to Mr. Lewison why my IQ score was so high, but I'll tell you. Mr. Lewison had told us the Friday before that on Tuesday the entire school year was having IQ testing. It was long before the Internet; I went to the Westminster Public Library, which housed one of London's largest medical libraries. I had been there several times to consult manuals about snail anatomy (*Playboy* to a snail lover). The library had a ledger-sized book, about two feet long, that contained all the age-adjusted state-approved IQ tests for UK schools. The first test I attempted from the book gave me an IQ of 105. I spent the entire weekend going through those tests again and again; by Sunday night I was averaging above 120. The IQ test Mr. Lewison gave us was identical to one in the book. One mystery solved.

It would take 34 years for me to solve the mystery of moving snails, but from age 11 on, I was obsessed by why things move. Science, I now realize, never discovers new things but only uncovers the secrets of nature. The patterns of movement had been established in the brains of my snails long before I studied them. But I'll tell you that experimenting—being a scientist—is the coolest thing in the world. Every day is an adventure into the unknown.

FROM WANDERING POND SNAILS TO MOTIONLESS WORMS

Clad in an immaculate white coat, Cheng Huang leans over a petri dish balanced on a microscope. He has a needle pinched tightly between his thumb and index finger. Staring down the microscope eyepieces, he watches a tiny worm on the palm-size petri dish. It wiggles across the nutrient-rich agar. He picks up the next petri dish. This worm lies still. With the needle tip he carefully prods the motionless worm. It curls in response—it is not dead. Soon it will die and not respond to the prod of the needle. For these worms and the 1,400 others in the experiment, just as for humans, movement defines life. Stillness is death.

The worms, Cheng and his colleagues discovered,[1] have specific genes that predetermine their transition from wriggling freely, to prod responsive, to still death. Genes program the transition of these simple worms from madly wriggly infant worms to still dead ones. The worms follow a genetic road map that charts the frenzied movement of youth, to slowly aging, to death. These genes are mirrored in fish, horses, nonhuman primates and humans. Movement is a programmatic part of life, as natural as breathing.

DEATH RATTLE

My first internship as a third-year medical student was at a small regional hospital north of London. One night, a 92-year-old woman was brought into the emergency room in respiratory arrest. She was gaunt and white. Her skin was cool. She had no respiration and I could not feel a pulse. We were about to call her time of death when her left wrist flickered and her fingers twitched—a single tiny movement, nothing else. This was long before the HIV and hepatitis epidemics, and I quickly started mouth-to-mouth resuscitation. The lady came around. It was that tiny movement that defined her as being alive.

Studies document that people move with natural rhythms throughout their lives. Think of newborn babies thrashing their arms and legs. Scientists used to argue that frenetic and disordered baby movements were wasting energy.[2] The new thinking is different; these early thrashing, wild movements are the stimuli that the limbs need to develop and for the brain to learn how to control them.[3] In fact, in premature brain-injured babies with stunted early development, therapists use Kinesthetic Stimulation Therapy, in which they move the tiny limbs to force the brain to reconnect and thrash baby style.[4]

Most newborns begin to sit at six months, try to pull themselves up by nine months and walk by two years. In fact, children who do not meet these milestones require a second look from the medical teams. The progression of early movement is so intricately programmed that it is predictable.[5]

Recently I went to the post office to send some packages abroad. In line in front of me was an elderly couple; the man had a cane; the woman, a slow, wide gait. The man with the cane stood just as still as the white-haired woman beside him. As people were helped, the couple shuffled forward. In front of this quiet pair was a father who was constantly screaming at his son and daughter, aged about six and eight. They could not stand still, even for a minute. One knocked over a pile of forms. "Isabella!" her father shouted. Some might claim that these children were badly behaved, but those of us who are parents know that children just can't help it. As I have watched my own children grow up, I can attest to the constant, never-ceasing movement of the six-year-old and the progressive shift in activity levels as children age. Adults move less than children—consider parents sitting on the bleachers as their children play sports. Then we age and become slower still. Like the elderly couple in front of me in the post office line, we zip around less and become more careful and studied with our movements. And eventually, when we stop moving, death casts its shadow.[6]

From birth through death there is a predictable, programmed timetable of movement. We transition from the frenetic nature of childhood, to the organized movement of adulthood, through the stillness of aging. Movement is not only the essence of life; it is the rhythm that defines our stage of living. Is it any wonder that compressing a moving body into a chair for decade after decade does it harm?

MOVING HUMANS: SAPIENS SANS SEDENTARY

Homo sapiens evolved over 2 million years to the drumbeat of natural selection. Natural selection is the process whereby tiny modifications in the DNA result in the body performing better to create a selection advantage. If two people are being chased by a saber-toothed tiger, and one is genetically a tiny bit faster, that person will escape and live to procreate. The slower person lags behind and gets eaten—yum.

Over 2 million years, human beings evolved from knuckle-brushing apelike forms that lived in the forests of Africa to the upright *Homo sapiens* of today.

A LOVE STORY

As humans evolved from tree-climbing forest-dwelling apes, they left the forests. Imagine two girl apes. Stefanie is an oddity; she has a genetic mutation that causes her to have a straight, stiff spine and walk upright, whereas Zoe is a traditional back-bent knuckle walker. Zoe climbs and swings from tree to tree more adeptly than stiff-backed Stefanie. As a result, Zoe gets the best tree nest, the hottest guy-ape and the best food. But stiff-backed Stefanie, disgruntled and alone, stands taller than Zoe and sees that there is a world of swishing grasses beyond the forest. Off Stefanie goes, beyond the confines of the forest, in search of food. Since there are no other apes there, she finds food aplenty. The good news for us is that when stiff-backed Stefanie ventured onto the plains of Africa, she also spotted across the swishing grass stiff-backed, uprightly mobile Stan (who had the same stiff-back genetic mutation). It was love at first sight. Because both Stefanie and Stan had the stiff-back mutation, their baby apes got it too and stood tall. That is how one genetic mutation can dramatically impact movement. In case you think that this is a ridiculous example, there is, in fact, a human syndrome originally called Stiffman Syndrome and now called Stiff Person Syndrome (yes, really!) that can be accounted for by a gene mutation.[7]

The other thing we learn from stiff-backed Stefanie and Stan is the interplay between environment and genes. If Stefanie and Stan had stayed in the forest rather than venturing out onto the grass-swishing plains, unable to climb, they would have not eaten and would have become emaciated, infertile, and would have died. It was the availability of the plains plus the behaviors of Stefanie and Stan that took them out of the forest to make glorious love, nourish and explore.

The issue of how behavior, genes and environment interact is the new wave in science. I have described the stiff-back gene and how it propelled Stan into Stephanie's arms. Now imagine that a second gene comes into play, the risk-taker gene. If you are an ape swinging through the trees, having the risk-taker gene is a bad thing. You swing for a branch that is too far away, and kerplonk! You are ape jelly on the forest floor.

Let us now examine the risk-taker gene in Stefanie and Stan's four children—Jilly, Jonny, Bert and Beatrice—living on the plains. All four of them had the stiff-back gene and stand erect.

Jilly and Jonny do *not* have the risk-taker gene. One day they are playing in the plains and venture to the edge of the forest.

There they meet our old friend the tree-swinging forest ape, Zoe. "What are you guys doing out of the forest?" Zoe asks. "Apes belong in the forest. Come back and join the community." Jilly and Jonny see hordes of apes swinging through the forest. They have no risk-taker gene, and so they are genetically compliant. They follow Zoe into the forest. Their fate is sad. Because they have the stiff-back gene, they do not climb so well. Soon they are hungry and weak, and from far above in the forest canopy, Zoe watches them die. She has a mean smile on her face—for Zoe is genetically a conformist (no risk-taker gene) and resents anyone different from her.

In contrast, brother Bert and sister Beatrice have the risk-taker gene. They are explorers. Because they have this genetic defect, they never venture back to the forest edge—they are genetically programmed to explore. They go farther than their parents ever went, and slowly and surely they and then their children make their way out of Africa to the new world beyond. They and their progeny become the new humans. Again, if you think this is a ridiculous concept, genes have been identified that indeed predict participating in high-risk behaviors.[8] What is more fascinating is that similar brain genes predict whether a person will participate in active leisure activities in our modern chair-sentenced world.[9]

So here in this love story of stiff-backed Stefanie and Stan we see:

1. The power of genes to affect the human body
2. The importance of the environment in determining whether a gene defect causes life or death
3. The importance of genes that affect behavior
4. The importance of how two genes can interact with life-changing consequences

We have examined the effects of just two genes. Now imagine how 21,000 genes might interact—because that's how many we have.

STIFF-BACKED HUMANS WALKED
ACROSS THE EARTH

Early apes became early humans, so-called early *Homo*.[10] Early *Homo* evolved until they ceased to walk in a knuckle-dusting fashion and stood erect. The skeletons from the five Dmanisi skulls, from the Republic of Georgia, showed that these first *Homo*s were short, and their legs enabled them to walk for long distances as fully upright bipeds. As the newer humans became progressively more erect, they spread across the world over 2 million years, not in cars or by airplanes but on foot; the more they evolved, the farther they walked. The new world was filled by people who walked.

Over the 2 million years that the human body evolved to walk, so too the human brain evolved to control it. Human thinking evolved from the human brain. Thoughts flow and ebb, as do the sweeps of arms and legs; dynamic bodies are dynamic minds.

Humans evolved over 2 million years to cultivate their new world. They did this walking. They built social collectives. They built shelters for their children with their dynamic, strong bodies and creative, active minds. People farmed and trapped animals with ingenuity. The earliest and most profound inventions—fire, the wheel, iron smelting, bridge building, fortification and agriculture—were a result of active minds and bodies alike. Tool development was—the fossils whisper to us—initially focused on warheads and crude knives. You can imagine that the tribe that killed the most efficiently acquired the homes, possessions, food and tools of the victims—winning genes conquered losing ones.

As humans developed the greater agility, speed and dexterity necessary to be successful hunters and warriors, they also evolved the ability to tame and exploit the land around them.

Two skills developed simultaneously: agriculture and hunting.[11] Agriculture involved learning how to find edible fruits and vegetables, till the land, cultivate crops, harvest produce, and store and prepare it safely. All of this work was carried out manually, sometimes using animals. Hunting emerged as an efficient method for obtaining food and skins. Rudimentary tools became more complex. For example, spears tipped with flints soon became bows and arrows.

As the human brain evolved, more sophisticated strategies developed in both agriculture and hunting. Agriculturalists worked out which types of soil worked best for certain crops. Hunters developed strategies for killing animals with the greatest efficiency and safety; for example, massive fossil finds of animal bones demonstrate that early humans discovered that chasing bison over a cliff top was a simple way of gathering a great deal of meat and skin. All of this was done on foot.

Modern neuroscience has become intrigued by the idea that the brain evolved as human skills evolved. The brain is not a static mesh of electrical wires connecting one computer chip to another. Instead, there is abundant evidence that the human brain is constantly adapting to changes in stimuli.[12] The brain changes both its structure and its function based on environmental cues. Over 2 million years of human history, the brain evolved in response to its environment and to the movement of the people within it.[13]

ADVANCED BRAINS, ADVANCED PSYCHOLOGY

The science of psychology thrived in Russia from the beginning of the twentieth century. For example, Lev Vygotsky, who died in 1934, led a school of psychology that developed the idea that higher cognitive functioning in children could be advanced through physical play, practical activities and the influence of an encouraging social environment. The communist regime then began to use psychology as one of its methods for sculpting an obedient society.[14] Scientists took kittens (if you are a cat lover, skip the next few paragraphs) and reared them in dark boxes. After several weeks, they killed these kittens and examined their brains. They discovered that the visual cortex in the brain, which is the area associated with visual processing, had not developed. Later experiments with dark-reared kittens showed them to be blind at 15 to 20 weeks of age because the visual cortex cells were functionless.[15] The part of the brain that would normally handle images had not developed because the cats were kept in dark boxes all of their lives until their miserable deaths. These early experiments demonstrated how environment influences brain structure. More recently it was discovered that there are brain chemicals, so-called neuroplasticity factors, that force changes in brain structure. These structural changes are subsequently associated with changes in brain function; this is how the brain adapts to changing environments.[16]

The human being evolved to walk millions of years ago, and over this time, the human capacity to think evolved too. The human brain is designed to think while moving, just as our bodies are. Knuckle-dusting apes left the forests of Africa and evolved to walk more and more upright; their brains would have adapted as well. Maybe then it is not surprising to learn that if this dynamic moving human was pushed into a chair, not only would the body suffer but so too would the mind. Sports cars are designed to be driven. If you take a Ferrari and allow it to sit idle for decades, it will clog with gunk. The human body and mind, though far more sophisticated, are equally prone to gunk up. Tie a human into a chair, and it seizes up and dies.

NO CATS WERE HARMED IN THE WRITING OF THIS BOOK

Talking about cats . . . When I lived in Cleveland, one Sunday afternoon I received a frantic phone call. "Jim, I need help," my friend George said. "Come over," he begged. He gave me an address; it was an apartment in midtown. George was sitting on a sofa with a half-dead cat on his lap. He was trying to feed her milk from a tea cup. She could hardly move. The apartment was in disarray. The cat had upturned and destroyed everything movable. The sofa had been shredded.

George had been asked by his girlfriend to look after her cat while she went on an archaeological dig just north of Addis Ababa. He received his first phone call from her three weeks later when she asked about the cat. He had completely forgotten. The cat survived, but George's relationship with his girlfriend did not.

Ancel Keys, from the University of Minnesota, starved prisoners to examine the physiological effects of starvation. In 1944 he recruited 36 imprisoned conscientious objectors and then exposed them to 24 weeks of semistarvation.[17] At first, with human starvation, Keys noted a short period of high anxiety with a twitching in subjects' fingers and limbs. But then as starvation persisted, his subjects became more sedentary; they sat most of the day, and their spontaneous movements, gait and thought processing slowed. After six months of starvation, Keys observed his subjects during refeeding. The sitting stopped and the prisoners began to walk and think normally again.

The prisoners and the cat exhibited the classic starvation response. With starvation, there is an initial frenetic search for food. After a few days, though, the brain shuts down the body to conserve energy. Buffalo, lions, wolves, dogs, cats, rats and fish show the same behavior.[18] In humans and Cleveland cats alike, movement, food and survival are inexorably linked. We move to eat to live. Movement defines life. Read on, because sitting is death.

HOW EVOLVED ARE YOU?

How many of these activities have you done in the last week *on your legs?*

1. Built a home or at least a portion of it (DIY counts)
2. Eaten food you grew

3. Got together face-to-face with members of your community living within a mile (but not family members; e.g., local church)
4. Physically demonstrated or fought for a cause you felt to be important
5. Volunteered
6. Protected your children or loved ones from harmful, unhealthy environments
7. Made tools or garments
8. Socialized with real, breathing people
9. Cooked your own breakfast
10. Cooked your own lunch
11. Cooked your own dinner
12. Hunted (Internet bargain hunting does not count)
13. Gone to work under your own power (e.g., foot, skateboard, bike)

SCORING

Give yourself 1 point for each yes answer.

    10+:   Brilliant! Fully evolved!
    8–10: Excellent. Evolving nicely, keep going!
    4–7:   Evolutionarily challenged. Much more evolution to do.
    0–3:   Dear oh dear! *Homo sedentarius.*

Humans have only sat for about 200 years, since we urbanized and industrialized. It's obvious that as a species we are not designed for chairdom. And so the modern *Homo sedentarius* is idling, gunked up, stifled and sick. It is a common-sense argument, but where are the data? Is there science to confirm the evil of your chair?

When I first presented studies that sitting may be a critical trigger in obesity, one of the most senior scientists in the obesity field stood up in a packed scientific audience and screamed at me, "This is such garbage!" It amused me that he had to get out of his chair and stand in order to condemn the idea. At the time, my voice was alone. But over the last decade, evidence has grown faster than iPhone sales that sitting all day is lethal.[19]

Over the next few chapters, I'll try to convince you that sitting causes an ABC of illnesses so haunting that you will start to despise your chair. Furthermore, I'll uncover the depth of data that demonstrates how sedentariness connects to sluggish brain function and wandering thoughts—there is a reason you surf the Internet midafternoon: your mind has been rendered sluggish by your body.

The true cost of the sitting disease is even greater than the litany of medical illnesses. Most at stake is your sense of well-being. We all have a capacity for happiness. Sitting somehow suppresses it. Sitting is more dangerous than smoking, kills more people than HIV and is more treacherous than parachuting. We are sitting ourselves to death. How did no one notice?

2

FEED ME, MOVE ME

ENERGY SUPPLIES ARE OFTEN USED TO DESCRIBE A PERSON: for example, "he has tons of energy," "I've got no energy today," "I am wiped out." This intrigued Antoine Lavoisier, a French physiologist and economist, 200 years ago, and he set out to understand the energy of life. As a starting point, he took a hapless guinea pig and popped it in a container of ice. He calculated that the energy burned by the guinea pig equaled the heat it was generating and that this was equivalent to the carbon dioxide it produced. Death, Lavoisier discovered as the guinea pig breathed its last breath, is when the energy of life ceases. This life energy, he concluded, was not an intangible religious essence but a measurable chemical entity definable by the amount of carbon dioxide a living being produces.[1] The guinea pig, you may be pleased to hear, had his revenge in a very French style: Lavoisier was beheaded in 1794, in the French revolution—*trés miserable!*

A pair of American army doctors, Wilbur Atwater and Francis Benedict, read Lavoisier's work and wanted to know if human life force—human energetics—was similar to guinea pig energetics. In 1902 Atwater and Benedict built an apparatus that resembled a prison cell.[2] They put a human volunteer inside and measured the amount of carbon dioxide he produced.

The heat he produced equaled the amount of carbon dioxide he exhaled. Thereafter, we began to understand how people burn energy.

CALORIE BURN

There are three ways people burn energy: basal metabolic rate, thermic effect of food and activity thermogenesis. A little additional energy can also be burned through stress or medications.

Your basal metabolic rate is the rate you burn energy for core body functions and is measured at complete rest without food. It accounts for about 60 percent of daily energy expenditure in a sedentary person. Nearly all of its variability is accounted for by body size—or, more precisely, lean body mass. The bigger a person, the greater his or her basal metabolic rate. The thermic effect of food is the energy expended in response to a meal—many people feel hot after eating a big meal. They are experiencing the energy expenditure associated with digestion, absorption and fuel storage. The thermic effect of food (the energy you burn converting foods into the body's metabolic fuel) accounts for about 10 percent of daily energy needs and does not vary greatly among people.

The remainder of human energy expenditure is from activity—activity thermogenesis. If you sit all day, your activity thermogenesis is almost zip. If you are always running about, your activity thermogenesis is high.

Activity thermogenesis can be subdivided into exercise and nonexercise activity thermogenesis (NEAT). Overall, for two adults of similar size, daily energy expenditure varies by as much as 2,000 calories. As noted, basal metabolic rate is largely accounted for by body size, and the thermic effect of food is small. Hence, activity thermogenesis must vary by approximately 2,000 calories per day.

If activity thermogenesis varies by 2,000 calories a day, is it because of exercise or is it because of NEAT?

Exercise is defined as "bodily exertion for the sake of developing and maintaining physical fitness"—for example, sports or visiting the gym.[3] The vast majority of people do not participate in exercise, and so, for them, exercise calories are zero. Even for the minority of people who do exercise, for most of them, exercise accounts for 100 calories per day. This is evident to anyone who has toiled hard on an exercise machine and looks at the display to see that only 200 calories have been expended. If this person exercises three times a week, they will exercise away 600 calories, which averages out to less than 100 calories per day. Thus, for the vast majority of people, daily routines—nonexercise activity thermogenesis (NEAT) calories—explain why an active person can expend 2,000 calories a day more than an inactive person of the same size.

NEAT is the energy expenditure of all physical activities other than volitional sporting-like exercise. It includes all those activities that render us vibrant, unique and independent beings, such as dancing, going to work or school, shoveling snow, playing the guitar, swimming or taking a walk. NEAT is expended every day and in every way and can most easily be classified as work NEAT and leisure NEAT.

NEAT CALORIES AT WORK AND PLAY

Overall, your job is the major predictor of NEAT. Active work can expend 2,000 calories per day more than a sedentary job. If your job is completely chair-bound, as it is for most Americans, you burn 300 NEAT calories per workday. If your job is upright, such as a homemaker or shop assistant, you can burn 1,300 NEAT calories/workday. If your job is physically strenuous, you can expend 2,300 NEAT calories/workday.[4]

Variability in leisure activities also accounts for substantial variability in NEAT. To understand to what degree leisure activities influence NEAT, 24 volunteers came to the lab. First we asked them to emulate their TV watching at home; this could involve using the remote or turning the pages of the TV listings, but mostly it involved sitting motionless.[5] Energy expenditure barely budged over resting values. Next the volunteers were asked to stay sitting but deliberately fidget by writing or knitting, for example. This pushed up their calories, but not a great deal (5 percent). We then asked our volunteers to stand completely still (not a big calorie burner: 10 percent). Finally, we wanted to understand how people burned calories while standing in a natural way, as they would at home, and so we asked our volunteers to emulate activities they typically did at home while standing. One man brought in his laundry to fold. One woman brought in a life-size toy cat; she repeatedly tripped over it in the lab. "This is what happens at home," she said. These types of activities almost *double* metabolic rate while standing and moving. But as soon as people walked gently at 2 mph, they *tripled* their calorie burn.

Compared to being at complete rest, watching TV burns 5 calories per hour, folding laundry 100 calories per hour and going for a stroll 200 calories per hour.[6]

The modern mechanization of everyday tasks has resulted in fewer NEAT calories compared with performing the same tasks manually.[7] Take four everyday tasks: by *not* walking to work, *not* climbing stairs and *not* manually washing clothes and dishes, we have lost an average of 111 NEAT calories per day. We all recognize, in addition, that there are many other chair-based activities that have displaced NEAT ones.

Say that I return home from work at 5 p.m. and watch television in a stupefied state, sitting, until I go to bed at 11 p.m. For these six hours, I will expend about 30 calories. Now consider that I flick the NEAT switch. In this incarnation, I return home and become aware of the unpainted bedroom and the ungathered leaves in the yard and decide to undertake these tasks. The total increase in NEAT can be 1,000 calories if I am busy all evening long.

For any given activity, the number of calories burned is the combination of how arduous the activity is multiplied by the time you do it for. A 30-minute exercise class may burn 200 calories, but an entire evening raking leaves (5 p.m. through 11 p.m.) may burn 1,000 calories. Sex may be arduous, but if it only lasts three minutes, it is not a big calorie burner! Thus, my choice of evening activity makes a big difference in NEAT.

To summarize, nonexercise activity thermogenesis—NEAT, the calorie burn of your daily routine—varies by as much as 2,000 calories a day. This is because some jobs are far more calorie burning than others and because leisure activities range from almost complete rest to those that are highly energized. Low NEAT is linked to weight gain, diabetes, heart attacks and cancer. But more important, if you have low NEAT—sitting disease—it means that you are not doing "stuff." A chair sentence is a low NEAT existence.

IF PEOPLE WHO SIT BURN FEWER CALORIES, ARE THEY MORE LIKELY TO GAIN BODY FAT?

I had long been interested in obesity—perhaps harking back to when I was 12 and suffered at the hands of a boy called Stone. Stone shoved my head down a toilet—for being fat. I was prone to obesity—even as a toddler I was endearingly called "Puffer." Perhaps it was my Jewish mother's overfeeding, perhaps it was genetic wiring. In addition, I was prone to stress eating. As my head lifted from the toilet bowl and I got up off my knees, I decided that I did not want to have obesity.

Obesity is an epidemic with catastrophic consequences already.[8] Obesity affects not only every organ system and body part, but also a patient's self-esteem.[9] My patients think about their obesity and the discrimination they feel approximately five times every hour.[10] Not only does obesity result in patients experiencing medical issues, discrimination and negative feelings; the financial costs are staggering. Obesity alone raises annual per capita medical costs in the United States by more than $3,000 per person, and if that person also has diabetes (which goes hand-in-hand with obesity), we are talking $10,000 per year per person.[11]

When I first came to Mayo Clinic as a medical student, I sought out the obesity experts. One way to escape a curse is to break it, and I wanted to find the cause of obesity. There I met Michael Jensen, a lean, brown-haired investigator with a pickax-dry sense of humor. He possessed what many scientists crave—the ability to distill vats of information into a conclusive concept. His colleague, Norm Eberhardt, was a tall, bearded genius whose liberalism harked back to his training in California. His understanding of humanity—he once had been slated to be a concert pianist—gave his biological insights meaning.

The three of us pondered the dream experiment to understand the cause of obesity. It is recognized that some people are more prone to obesity than others despite living in the same environments and having similar home situations. What is it about some people that makes them obese? What is the secret sauce in lean people that keeps them thin? The modern environment may be obesogenic—prone to inducing obesity—but some people survive it.

We figured that if we could overfeed a whole group of people the same number of excess calories, we could examine why some people are predisposed to gain body fat while others are resistant to fat gain. We realized that for this study to have relevance, all of our volunteers would need to continue with their normal jobs. This type of experiment had never been done before. We would overfeed free-living people and measure their fat gain. If we measured all aspects of their calorie burn, we would be able to discover how some people remain thin at the same time that others gain fat. With this experiment, we were on the hunt for the root cause of obesity.

Not many people wanted to be overfed (go figure!). We needed 16 people for the statistics; after 18 months, we had 15. My boss was asking awkward questions—I had been in the lab for almost two years and had not published a word. Despite radio and TV advertisements, I could not get the sixteenth person to participate, so I loosened my belt and became the final overfeeding volunteer myself.

THE GREAT GORGING EXPERIMENT

Starting in 1996, all 16 of us ate all of our food for ten weeks in Mayo's Metabolic Research Unit. Every single food item was weighed out by the gram. Sometimes I would get a piece of bread with a corner cut off, or two-thirds of an egg, or a tomato with a piece missing. The metabolic kitchen knew everything I was eating. For the first two weeks, I was fed exactly the amount of food that was necessary to keep my body weight rock steady. Then the fun began. For the next eight weeks, I was overfed by 1,000 calories above my needs. Eating an excess of 1,000 calories a day is not as arduous as you might think. It is the equivalent of an extra Big Mac and a shake spread over a day.

All the volunteers were overfed in the same way—1,000 calories a day above and beyond what they normally ate. For all of us, this went on seven days a week for eight weeks, and so everyone ate an excess 56,000 calories above their normal needs. Three times a day, we came to the research unit, ate and then went back to our normal lives. Since we were careful to have recruited "normal" people, gym goers were not allowed. (Only 15 percent of Americans regularly go to a gym, and so they're not normal!) As volunteer followed volunteer through this belly-splitting protocol, I realized that the secret to the whole project was Martha.

Martha was our research cook. She was five feet tall and broad. She had a smile the size of the Atlantic Ocean but a will stronger than steel. Martha had been a professional chef and, judging by the twinkle in her eye, a successful one. She could entice you to eat far beyond your stomach's capacity just with a smile—at least most of the time. One night I was on the research unit and heard raised voices from the dining room. I ran there to see Martha standing in front of a six-foot volunteer from the overfeeding study. "Drink it," she said. She was ordering him to drink the greasy juice that had come off a hamburger he had eaten. "No way," he replied. "Drink it!" she said. The smile had been drained from her voice like tea from a twice-used tea bag. Voices rose further. "No, I won't," the man said. "Yes, you will!" Martha ordered. Eventually, shaking slightly, the towering volunteer raised the dinner plate to his lips and drank the juice from the hamburger. Martha saw me and a smile jumped back on her face. "Dr. Levine said you have to get every calorie," she reminded the man.

All 16 volunteers were overfed by an *exact* excess of 56,000 calories—I am certain!

Before and after Martha's gourmet gorge, we performed meticulous measurements of our volunteers' energy stores and calorie burn. Every one of Martha's extra 1,000 calories per day had to be accounted for. An extra calorie could be stored, burned off or pooped out. To assess my body's fuel stores and how they changed with overfeeding, I went through computed tomography (CT) scans, X-ray absorbance scans and biopsies of my body fat before and after the 56,000-calorie gorge. Similarly, to assess my calorie burn before and after the overfeeding period, I had respiratory measurements at rest, after eating and walking. I collected buckets of urine, and in case I pooped out the extra calories, I had to collect my stool too.

Wherever those extra 1,000 calories a day went, we'd find them! Some of our research volunteers were followed into toilets; we listened through the wall to ensure that they were not vomiting. By the time the experiment was over, we had collected buckets of urine and tubs full of feces. We drew blood samples with a zest greater than in a Brad Steiger vampire novel. We had freezers full of body fat samples (for the longest time I was known as "the fat guy"). One of our volunteers showed me a journal she wrote. In it I was described as something between Attila the Hun, Dracula and Gordon Ramsey.

The Great Gorging Experiment took a total of three years to complete, during which time I was berated by my boss—all that time and nothing to show. All the data were blinded, so we knew nothing of the results until the final urine samples were measured at the University of Cambridge—they had specialized mass spectrometers we didn't have at Mayo—at the very end of the study. I remember sitting in front of a constantly crashing computer in Cambridge and hitting the enter key. As if the Almighty were teasing me, the computer crashed again—the amount of data we had gathered was overwhelming. I tried again. And then before me shone the answer to obesity—why some people are more prone to gain fat while others stay thin.

WHAT WAS THE SECRET? WHY DO SOME PEOPLE GAIN MORE FAT THAN OTHERS?

Every one of our 16 volunteers had received an excess 56,000 calories—Martha had ensured that. Some had placed almost every single calorie into their fat stores—they'd gained 14 pounds of fat (there are 3,500 calories in a pound of fat). I indeed fell into this category. Others in the experiment, however, burned off all of Martha's excess food. How had they done it? How can a person be overfed by an excess 1,000 calories per day and not gain a pound of fat? The answer is NEAT—nonexercise activity thermogenesis—the calories that people burn moving about their day *when they are not sitting.*[12]

People who have the ability to switch on their NEAT movement do not gain fat with overfeeding; they stay slim. People who stay seated when they overfeed, and don't switch on their NEAT movement, deposit all of the extra calories into body fat.

Some people have a powerful NEAT switch—when they overeat, as we all do periodically, they switch *on* their NEAT and burn off the extra pounds. Other people don't have this capacity—they store every extra calorie they consume in their fat stores.

NEAT is the pivot to obesity. I have a question for you. Have you ever gained 5 pounds (or more) . . .

> . . . after a vacation?
> . . . with a job change?
> . . . when you went to college?
> . . . when you got married (a big issue for men)?
> . . . after a pregnancy?
> . . . during a stressful time in your life?

Most people answer yes to at least one of these questions. (I answered yes to all these possibilities—I even gained 10 pounds during my wife's first pregnancy!) But my next question to you is this: Did you lose the weight again afterward?

Imagine Roxanne—25 and slim—who has the physiological makeup to unconsciously flick *on* her NEAT switch. Roxanne takes a holiday to Miami and gains 5 pounds, but afterward, her NEAT switch is activated, and she burns off the extra calories and is back to her normal weight. Then she takes a new job, which leads to a 15-pound weight gain. Her NEAT switch turns on; then she loses the weight. Then she gains 20 pounds with her first baby—with her NEAT switch *on*, she loses the 20 pregnancy pounds. A decade later, Roxanne is the same weight as she was at 25.

Now imagine Celeste—25 and slim—but she, like most Americans, does *not* have a powerful NEAT switch. Celeste has the same exposures as Roxanne; she goes to Miami, gets a new job and has a baby. Without the NEAT switch, a decade later she weighs 40 pounds more.

We had found the secret. Those people who do not have a NEAT switch remain sitting in response to overfeeding and are predisposed to obesity. Obesity is the consequence of sedentariness, a sedentariness that is so profound that it kills the body's capacity to burn off extra fuel.

HOW SOME PEOPLE STAY THIN

My mother used to read me a book when I was a child called *Fattypuffs and Thinifers* by André Maurois. It depicted a cartoon society comprised of portly persons and super-thin people. The book read: "Lazy and amiable. Fattypuffs are like overstuffed chairs and large, squashy pastries. Thinifers on the other hand are a lean and energetic bunch." These were clichéd images, but our overfeeding studies affirmed the notions that some people are naturally prone to develop obesity. Other people are naturally lean.

We had discovered what it is about energetic Thinifers and how they stay lean; they switch on their NEAT switches, and their increased NEAT burns off any extra food they happen to eat. People with obesity do *not* activate NEAT when they overfeed and as the years pass, their weight increases.

At this point I could have shrugged my shoulders and said to my patients battling obesity, "You were right all along. People with obesity have slow metabolism—low NEAT." But what good would that have done my patients?

The overfeeding study gave the scientific community fascinating insight into the biology of obesity (low NEAT) but the real question had to be, how can NEAT be exploited to help the three in ten Americans who are seriously trying to lose weight?[13] We needed more information. We did not understand *why* people with obesity have low NEAT. To answer this question, we entered the enticing world of underwear—better still, *magic* underwear.

MAGIC UNDERWEAR

In order to look within the lives of people with obesity and understand why they fail to burn off NEAT calories, a technology was needed to measure the ins and outs of daily living. Since most people wear underwear on most days, I figured that if sensors were attached to people's underwear, I could sneakily measure what they were up to day in and day out. Having gone through several career-counseling sessions while at school, underwear design was never discussed. Nonetheless, I was ready to take the plunge. After several unsuccessful visits to underwear stores, though, I realized that I needed help. Enter electronic underwear designers extraordinaire: Paulette and Paul.

Paul had been a senior engineer at IBM. Retired, he was now looking for something meaningful to do in his twilight years. I invited him to join the lab "to develop anti-obesity technology," I told him. Underwear design was not on his horizon. His magic underwear design collaborator was a young scientist who had previously worked for The Gap; she was named Paulette.

They got to work. I would come into the lab and see Lycra spandex creations cut into the most unusual shapes with wires shooting out of them. The Mayo computers frequently blocked my searches for different underwear styles (if you look, the variety is impressive). Paul, in his 60s, and Paulette, in her 30s, would be engaged in heated debates about male and female bodies and the hole sizes necessary to accommodate them. What they came up with was bizarre but effective. The holes enabled all biological functions to continue as normal. In the meantime, the sensors we attached to the underwear allowed us to measure all postures and movements of our volunteers continuously.

Magic underwear, for the first time, enabled us to track not only how individuals move throughout the day and night but also their body positions every half second.[14] Especially at night, people contort themselves into the most unusual positions! The good news is that these contortions do not appear to last for very long—most for fewer than three minutes. Suffice it to say, for the first time in history, we were able to map *everything* that a person does day and night for weeks.

We recruited an army of fairly typical people willing to give up their usual underwear for ours; all had desk jobs, and none went to the gym. They put on the magic underwear, and the data came in.

What we discovered was astonishing. People with obesity who lived in the same environment as people who are lean, *sit more*—a lot more. Sitting caused the low-NEAT calorie burn of obesity. It was not food that explained the differences between lean and obese people, because we controlled the types of food and the diets were balanced—Martha cooked again. People with obesity *sat* 2 hours and 15 minutes more a day than lean volunteers. Obesity, we discovered, was the archetypal sitting disease. People who are chair sentenced the most are the most likely to have obesity.

After a decade of research, we had proved that obesity was a chair addiction. The chair is fattening.

CAN A PIECE OF FURNITURE HARM YOU?

The notion that a piece of furniture can harm you took me back to my internship days in Barnet General Hospital, north of London. As a surgical intern, I got used to the so-called 1 a.m. granny dump. If midnight is when elderly relatives call their children, 1 a.m. is when the children dump granny in the emergency room and drive off: "We can't leave our kids at home by themselves" is the typical excuse.

In one such case, a large elderly woman in her late 80s was left in the emergency room. I was on-call. She was an archetypal granny: blue-rinse hair, a sweet, toothless smile and bad breath. She also smelled as if she had not bathed in quite some time. Her main complaint was severe back pain.

With the help of a nurse, we rolled her onto her side so I could look at her back. Most of her back was a red, weeping bedsore, so raw that she had left large bloodstains on the white hospital sheet. At her home, the patient's bed had worn through her skin because she never moved.

The blue-rinse granny and her bedsores explain how a simple piece of furniture can be lethal. Good-quality sleep is essential for health.[15] However, the overuse of furniture—a bed in this case—can cause harm.

Same too with the chair: There is nothing innately harmful about a chair unless you sit on it too much.

THE SCIENTIFIC COMMUNITY

The world press was interested in how sitting caused obesity, but convincing the scientific community was more challenging. The first conference I lectured at after the sitting-causes-obesity discovery was in Atlanta in 2000. Scientists had heard about what we were doing, and the lecture hall was crowded. I realized that since sitting disease was a new concept, I would need to represent it in a way that pushed back traditional boundaries. I wore a wireless microphone and paced around the lecture hall as I spoke. After I finished my lecture, it was time for questions.

One of the most senior professors in the field, let's call him Professor Smallbrain, stood up. "This sitting disease is all nonsense," he began. He went on, "Dr. Levine, how can you have the audacity to claim that sitting down causes harm?" For more than a decade I'd read and admired Professor Smallbrain's papers, and now a hero of mine was rebuking me before my peers. He went on and on and on. In his screaming fit, he used the words "disgrace" and "shameful." I don't remember much more.

The beating I took from the scientific community had only just begun. I returned to work, but the word was out. Colleagues did not answer correspondence, and my scientific papers drew spiteful and badly argued critiques.

Next, I went to Orlando to deliver a plenary lecture. Shortly after returning from this lecture, I was summoned to see my boss. A scientific competitor of mine—let's call him Dr. Micromind— had written to Mayo; in his opinion, I was psychiatrically unsound or even potentially deranged. He wrote: "I have so long respected Jim's work, but I'm worried that he is gone off the rails."

My boss was worried and sent me to see a psychiatrist. The psychiatrist saw the letter from Micromind and knew it for precisely what it was. While I sat there, he called five of my colleagues;

he asked each, "Is Dr. Levine in your opinion of sound mind?" The calls were brief. All of my colleagues concurred that I was sane, and I returned to work. A week after this event, I received a letter from the president of the scientific society I had given the plenary lecture to. "Your work is revolutionary. Good luck," he wrote.

But this episode shook me. Having your sanity questioned is strange. In science, our ideas are the air we breathe. To have one scientist scream that my work was "nonsense" and another claim I was insane unsettled me—for a while. My friends said my detractors were jealous. But I understood better. It was a conspiracy. Obviously, The Chairman had paid off these scientists to conspire against me and shame me. It is not paranoia if you are right.

It was time to get back to work. The foundation for a new science had been laid: lethal sitting was born.

LAB APPLICATION QUESTIONNAIRE

Do you want to join our lab? Please complete the following knowledge-based evaluation.

Running for a bus burns more calories than sitting — True/False

Tripping over your cat (imaginary or real) burns more calories than sitting — True/False

Black Friday shopping at Wal-Mart burns more calories than sitting — True/False

Dancing at a party burns more calories than sitting — True/False

Climbing trees burns more calories than sitting — True/False

Folding laundry burns more calories than sitting — True/False

Chewing gum burns more calories than sitting — True/False

Jumping out of your chair burns more
calories than sitting   True/False

If you answered True to all of these questions, welcome to the
NEAT lab. You are ready to be freed from your chair sentence.

3

THE BRAIN STRAIN

I ACQUIRED MY FIRST LAB THROUGH SQUATTER'S RIGHTS. There was an abandoned specimen-cutting room by the chapel in an old part of the hospital at Mayo. The room had been used for decades to prepare samples for microscopic analysis. One morning, I was the attending covering the Hospital Nutrition Service when I noticed a pile of discarded laboratory equipment in a corridor. That night, I moved it all into the empty specimen room. Voilà! I had my own lab. It was better than getting my first apartment—it was like having a personal space rocket to take me to places no one else had ever been.

Over a year or so, grants accumulated, and I slowly disposed of the discarded equipment and brought in equipment that worked. In one part of the lab, which used to be an office, I built a contraption to measure sedentariness, activity and calorie burn in animals ranging in size from rats to worms. There were several mishaps. To validate the equipment, it was necessary to burn known amounts of butane within the system. I failed to realize that the plastic I had used to build the animal cages had a low melting temperature; but that was what the sprinkler system was for. Anyway, it wasn't the first lab I had blown up.

As time went by, several phenomenal neuroscientists collaborated with me to examine the brain circuits of sedentary behavior. Catherine Kotz was the first neuroscientist I came to work with. Our working relationship started off in the worst way possible. Shortly after the Great Gorging study was published in 1999, I was sitting in a coffee shop in Nairobi, where I was volunteering with the Red Cross, inching through email, when I saw a series of emails from the University of Minnesota. The first started politely: "Where are you?" The next was less polite: "Are you coming?" The third was cross: "Don't say you aren't showing up?" I was supposed to be teaching Professor Kotz's students 8,000 miles away at the University of Minnesota; I had forgotten.

I pled ignorance, begged forgiveness and asked for a second chance. A month later I was sitting in a University of Minnesota classroom awaiting Cathy Kotz. From the tone of her emails, I expected a dragon. When I heard a rapid click-click-click coming down the corridor outside, I swallowed and dried my sweaty hands. No dragon. Instead entered a young, elegant woman wearing bright red stiletto shoes and a dark blue suit. Her demeanor showed potential reconciliation. She is one of America's leading neuroscientists.

Over the next few years, Dr. Kotz visited my Mayo lab frequently. She used our animal measurement facility to monitor animal movements and their calorie burn in response to changes in brain chemistry. To change the brain's chemical neurotransmitters, she would sedate a rat and advance a long, thin needle deep into its hypothalamus at the center of its brain. Amazingly, this neither hurt nor harmed the animal. She could then instill minuscule chemical doses into the hypothalamus and measure whether animal sedentariness could be reversed.

The part of the brain she was fascinated by was the paraventricular nucleus of the hypothalamus, which in the rat is smaller than a period.[1] One neurochemical that had just been discovered, orexin, wakes you up from sleep. The orexin-deficient dog has narcolepsy—randomly falling asleep without warning (not the best guard dog!). Sleep is the time where you have least movement, so orexin was interesting to us as a neurochemical that might help get people moving.

Cathy took a group of 24 rats and inserted needles into the center of their brains; half she injected with orexin. The others received water injections. It was instantly obvious which ones received the neurochemical. The animals that had received orexin raced around the cage as if they were late for a meeting, whereas the animals that received water injections snoozed from time to time and occasionally wandered around their cages. Discovery is the cocaine of science. We published our first paper in 2002, and Cathy at last forgave me.

Experiment followed experiment, and other scientific groups dived in. It was indisputable that there are neurochemicals that control whether you sit or walk; orexin was one. It changes the way you look at the world: Next time you are sitting at a bus stop or in a café, look at the people around you. Some will be still, but others will shuffle and fidget. These are not random movements but are the result of brain "move-it" factors.

The rats Cathy had injected with neurochemicals enabled us to begin understanding how the brain controls sedentariness versus movement. Because we were injecting chemicals directly into the "master control" center of the brain, we could be certain that these mediators of NEAT were impactful. It was clear from her experiments that brain chemistry can drive a rat to be either a couch potato or superactive. But we needed to know more: Can these non–exercise-type movements impact body weight and obesity?

To take the next step, I needed a neuroscientist willing to dive deeper. Colleen Novak, an experienced neuroscientist from Georgia, called, wanting to work with us. She sent her curriculum vitae, but she had no experience in obesity energy research. Two weeks later I received a phone call; the woman at the other end began, "You have to hire me. I'm telling you—I get it!" I invited Colleen to Rochester.

When I worked in Nairobi, I had a drink with Jane Goodall, the famed chimp scientist. Colleen had the same eyes—soft fire. She was the least experienced obesity scientist I ever hired, but her eyes burned as she spoke. She explained how she would take Cathy Kotz's animal work to the next level. Her plans were insanely ambitious. I hired her on the spot.

Over the next five years, Colleen discovered that there is a whole network of brain chemicals that sink us into our chairs or propel us out of them.

One afternoon I happened to be in Victoria Station in Mumbai, India, at 4 p.m. Thousands of people streamed through the station in the wet afternoon heat. Trains came in—bringing families into the city. Trains set out—taking workers home. The outward traffic was greater than the inward; as trains left the station, people hung out of doorless carriages. This is a metaphor for how non-exercise, spontaneous movements are controlled: Mumbai is the brain's hypothalamus, Victoria Station the paraventricular nucleus and India is the body. The train tracks are neurons that pass in and out. Neurotransmitter molecules ride these tracks back and forth.

Colleen not only explored the station and the tracks' destinations, she also discovered a host of chemicals—different types of passengers—that either propelled a rat to clamber about or to slouch in its recliner. Chemical followed chemical—Colleen marched on.

Colleen Novak had all the ingredients necessary to become a great scientist: intelligence, political awareness, "elbows" (the scientist's most important tool for nudging other scientists out of the way) and drive. I stood over her shoulder as she won her first federal grant from the National Institutes of Health. With skilled rat breeders, she launched a multigenerational rat breeding experiment to uncover whether the tendency to sit is hardwired into the obese rat's brain.

FAT RATS AND THINIFERS

In Colleen's study, generation after generation of rats were mated for obesity or leanness. Obese rats were mated with obese rats and lean rats with lean rats. Once Colleen had fat rats and Thinifers, she started to inject her chemicals into the center of their brains. She discovered that the brains of the obese rats had NEAT switches that were stuck in the OFF position. Regardless of the amount of move-it chemicals, these fat rats could not switch on their NEAT. They had a genetic wiring *not* to respond to move-it signals. Fat rats were wired for the couch (chair addicts with tails).

When Thinifer rats had their brains injected, in contrast, their NEAT switches flicked ON with ease; the lean rats almost leaped out of their cages and engaged in a frenzied dance of excited movement. Thinifers were built to move—they were so frenzied that they even spilled their food as they madly ate.

THE TALE (TAIL) OF MARATHON-RUNNING MUSCLE

Colleen and I were having a drink one day, and I spoke sacrilegiously. "Imagine that it is *not* the brain that controls sitting and movement." Her dark eyes darted at me and she frowned. "Like what then?" she asked. "Perhaps the muscle informs the brain," I suggested. If you go for a run, after a while your muscles feel tired. It is not your brain telling your muscles to feel tired. The tiredness signal comes from the muscles themselves. Perhaps it is true of sitting as well. Perhaps the sit signal comes from the muscle. Perhaps tired muscles signal the brain to sit. Imagine you are working hard in the fields or hunting; it makes sense that exhausted muscles tell your brain, "I need a break!"

Colleen looked at me. "Other scientists have studied genetically bred marathon-running rats," she said.[2] "Why don't we see if these rats are chair haters too? Perhaps the brains of marathon-running rats don't listen to the muscle signals to sit!"

Colleen called up the other group of scientists, and soon we had marathon-running rats in the lab plus their counterparts, genetically bred rats that loathed long-distance running. Colleen's test results were incredible. Marathon-running rats spontaneously darted around a cage, far more so than couch potato rats. Colleen discovered that the marathon runners' muscles are different; their muscles inform the brain to continuously keep moving. Genetic movers have muscles that stop them from sitting.

Conversely, the other animals that were genetically bred to hate marathon running mooched around their cages, nosing around for a TV remote control. They were sedentary sitters. It was clear that the sit-still circuit was not just in the brain but in the muscle too.[3]

I lived in Minnesota for 25 years, with four-month sub-zero winters, and learned a lot about heating systems. A heating system has a central thermostat that switches on the furnace when the house cools. In my house the central thermostat received information from temperature sensors located throughout the house. In the same way, NEAT is controlled primarily by the brain. Signals stream in from all over the body: the muscle, the fat and the senses. (If you are watching a gripping movie, you are unlikely to move. A bang may make you jump.) These signals inform the brain as to the current state of NEAT.

It appeared that a Thinifer is super-sensitive to "move-it" signals. When the Thinifer has sat for too long, the NEAT controller in the brain switches ON and fires a Get Up signal. The Thinifer fidgets and then jumps up and burns NEAT.

A person prone to obesity is less sensitive to "move-it" signals; the muscle is used to sitting, and a long movie does not prompt any Get Up signals, and so the chair sentence and obesity are perpetuated.

Other scientists from around the world became interested in the importance of sitting in obesity; sedentary science was taking off! People who are movers have brains firing "move-it" signals all the time, and their brains respond like crazy to those "move-it" signals. The brains of people who have a tendency toward obesity are nonresponsive to "move-it" signals. Thus, the brain is hardwired to make you move or seduce you to sit. But it is not just the brain that makes you a sitter. If you have sitter-type muscle, you'll sit more too. Sitting-predisposed brains may create sitting muscles because if you sit a lot, your muscles *become* sedentary.

Reading this, you may feel that your fate has been pre-determined—you are either a Thinifer or a person convicted to a lifelong chair sentence. Are chairaholics really *condemned* to a life of chairdom?

FROM RATS TO CATS

As mentioned in chapter 1, the adaptability of the brain was orig-inally shown in experiments in which cats locked in dark rooms showed different brain development compared to cats kept in the light. The environment influences the structure of the brain.

This may seem confusing if you argue that DNA is the blue-print for the brain's structure and thus brain structure should be fixed. But consider the heart. The heart's structure is determined by DNA too. If, however, a person exposes their heart to islands of ice cream, oceans of alcohol and vats of cholesterol, the heart, despite having good DNA, malfunctions. Conversely, a Tour de France cyclist with the same DNA has a heart that is efficient. In this example, DNA provides the basic structure of the heart, but its structure is not fixed—it responds well to being looked after and malfunctions if abused.

The same is true of a building. On the day it is opened, a well-constructed building may be glorious and beautiful. How-ever, if it is badly maintained and sits empty and uncared for, it will crumble and ruin. The human brain is similar; the DNA defines a structural blueprint. Interaction with the environment through sight, sound, smell, touch and taste shapes the brain's structure and function. The brain's wiring system is laid down based on the DNA blueprint, but it adapts substantially to the stimuli that the brain is exposed to. If you douse your brain in alcohol, it will eventually pickle. A person in France may have the same brain DNA structural blueprint as a person in China, but only one of them speaks French. If you sit all day unstimulated, your brain will fall into ruin.

How does the brain adapt to the environment? The brain's wiring system is a mesh of neurons. But rather than being made of copper, these wires are made from a material like chewing gum that curves, twists, separates and stretches. Neuroplasticity factors are responsible for the stretchiness of the neurons.[4] These neuroplasticity factors allow the brain's structure to change with the environment. Sit all day and your brain looks different from the brain of a mover.

If you sit for a long period, the brain becomes sedentary in structure and then ultimately in thought patterns—a seated body begets a sedentary mind. But the good news is, if a chairaholic takes the first step, gets up and walks, the brain, like a muscle, adapts. The walking brain fires new neuroplasticity factors, and over time the brain adapts to its owner's newfound propensity to walk. Because the brain is constantly adapting, it takes about three weeks for brain change to occur. A chairaholic can become a walker in three weeks. But watch out! A walker who begins to sit can just as easily become a chairaholic.

Over the last few generations, millions of brains have become sedated by sedentariness. Most people in the modern Western world are sitters. Just as the brain adapts to chairdom, so does the whole of society. If most people become sitters, the structure of society gradually adapts to become chair-based. No sidewalks are laid in new neighborhoods, offices and homes adapt so that sitting is the default body position, theater chairs become softer and wider, drive-throughs develop and shopping becomes a wrist action rather than a leg-based activity. Chicken or egg—did society make the sitters, or did sitters make the society? The answer: Both occurred.

We have created for ourselves a modern way of living that clashes with the way we're meant to be. We have converted from an ancient world of movers to a modern world of chair sloths. But it is not just our bottoms that have become wider; our brains have become sedated as well. However, we can reverse the chair sentence just as we once succumbed to it. You can adapt to survive. You can get up.

WIRED RIGHT

Six wiring blueprints for the human brain follow. Only one is wired as nature designed. Can you spot it?

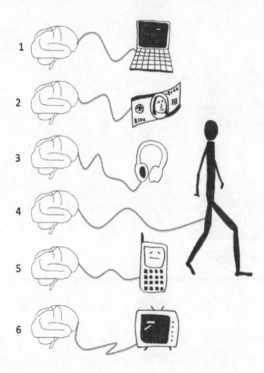

4

DESPITE YOUR CHAIR, YOU ARE AN INDIVIDUAL

IN MONTY PYTHON'S MOVIE *THE LIFE OF BRIAN*, BRIAN (THE Jesus character) stands before the assembled masses, spreads his arms and shouts, "Look, you've got it all wrong. You don't *need* to follow me. You don't *need* to follow *anybody*. You've got to think for yourselves. You're *all* individuals."

The crowd shouts back in unison, "Yes, we're all individuals."

Brian calls back, "You're all different."

The crowd replies, "Yes. We *are* all different."

Then someone puts up his hand and says, "I'm not!"

IT IS UNIMAGINABLE TO US today that a few hundred years ago, many people did not view themselves as individuals but as the property of others. If a person hated her master, she had no option to work for another employer, start her own business or engage in independent commerce. What happened to change that?

As with many social revolutions, the shift did not occur through a single act, moment or person. In the West, the idea of individuals being able to think for themselves and be independent of the control of their masters arose during the seventeenth century. Before then, masters, monarchs and church leaders had absolute power over their subjects by "divine right"—God selected the rulers and the rules. But a shift in thinking began with England's Glorious Revolution of 1688. A parliament was established to represent the people. With this sense of individual power arose the cultural movement called the Enlightenment. People started to understand their roles as individuals and their rights to make personal and even moral decisions for and about themselves.

During the Enlightenment, the superstars in society were not athletes or singers but intellectuals. Wherever he went, Jean-Jacques Rousseau, for example, was treated with similar adoration as Taylor Swift or LeBron James is treated today.

After the Enlightenment, individuals had the right to live more as they chose. People started to farm independently and aggregated in self-governing towns and villages. Communities popped up where resources permitted—for instance, in areas where the soil was fertile or around local resources, such as lumber. Service providers, such as cobblers, tailors and doctors, established themselves in larger, financially successful communities; people living in smaller communities traveled by foot or horse to access the service providers. Society grew. At this point in our story, people were active from sunrise to sunset, resting occasionally on chairs, *but* they had the freedom to move to where the economic climate was brightest.

About 250 years ago, the invention of steam engines and mechanization changed the landscape. The Industrial Revolution began and precipitated the greatest change in human living since we'd left the forests in central Africa 2 million years before.

THE INDUSTRIAL REVOLUTION— FACTORIES SWIPE OUR LEGS

We often assume that events in history occurred more slowly than do current events. However, the Industrial Revolution, which marked one of the most profound changes in the human way of life, occurred over only 50 years or so, beginning around 1760.

The Industrial Revolution involved changing from using manual methods to complete tasks to using machines. It began in Britain. Charles Dickens wrote about London in this period; he described the industrialists' enormous wealth but also urban poverty, child labor and workhouses. The steam engine allowed for automation, and factories sprang up across the manufacturing sector. People moved from agricultural communities to the cities, where the jobs were. Power sources changed as well, from oxen to coal. By the 1850s the Industrial Revolution had spread to the United States and Europe. The relocation of people from the fields into industrial cities was unstoppable; so too was their descent to chairdom.

A TALE OF THREE CITIES

1. Phoenix, Arizona

It is 6 a.m. and the sun has just risen over the red rock of Piestewa Peak. The sun's power is intense; it sears my skin as I climb. Two-thirds of the way up the mountain is a clearing covered by small pebbles. The original Native American people who sat here ruled over a green valley, irrigated by 135 miles of hand-dug canals feeding off the Salt River. Below me I see the morass of intersecting streets and avenues that is the modern city of Phoenix.

Concrete is far and wide. To the east, Phoenix transitions seamlessly to the city of Scottsdale—with its own plumage of high-rises and a dense array of homes. The buildings are the colors of sand and gray concrete, and the streets teem with cars. The metropolitan complex of 6 million is not entirely devoid of green; the cities have planted trees and built parks. One hundred fifty years ago, Phoenix was an agricultural oasis; now it is a modern metropolis.

We cannot imagine the lifestyle of people two centuries ago, who lived in this valley before the concrete came. We can only perceive that which is immediately in our context and imagine that which is told to us by the living. We have no memory of what it was to live a manual leg-based life. Concrete, chair-based living is all that we know.

2. Kinshasa, Democratic Republic of Congo

In 2010 I was visiting a small community of people who had been rejected by their society in the Democratic Republic of Congo. They lived ten miles to the east of the Kinshasa airport. All had AIDS and had been thrown out of their homes by husbands, children or wives. Somehow they found each other and banded together to form a community.

The community was cohesive, self-supporting and successful. The members, as they referred to themselves, got healthcare from Doctors Without Borders and received HIV drugs for free from the Global Fund. Each person was allocated a strip of land, about 12 yards by 2, to farm. About half of this strip of land was necessary to sustain the person; the remainder of the crop was sold to benefit the community. This community was so successful financially, compared to the slum areas of Kinshasa, that people without HIV infection pretended to have it in order to be admitted.

One evening I found myself watching the sun set over Kinshasa with this community of 24 survivors. We sat on plastic chairs around a tree, drinking Coca-Cola and Fanta from glass bottles and chatting. The community members had worked all day farming their land. They were exhausted. As the sun began to set, it was time for a break.

The community had a self-appointed director who was referred to as Madame Directrice. Soon after the group convened, she lifted her hands over her head and started to click her fingers. Others in the group stopped talking and began to click their fingers as well. (Of course I joined in.) Then one member shuffled away and returned soon after with bottles of antiretrovirals, which were passed around the circle from hand to hand; everyone took their HIV medications together. Then there was silence, and Madame Directrice formally welcomed me. Through my interpreter, Papa John, Madame Directrice asked me to tell my story. I began to explain my journey to Kinshasa from Minnesota. Madame Directrice interrupted me. She wanted me to tell a story, not *my* story. I thought for a moment. The first thing that popped into my head were stories my grandfather, Poppa, used to tell me. They were about a group of children called Cry-a-lot, Moan-a-lot and Laugh-a-lot. I told the Kinshasa community the story of how Moan-a-lot complained one day about the ceaseless rain (remember, I am from England!) while at the same time Laugh-a-lot jumped shoeless in the puddles.

When I was done, Madame Directrice pointed to another member of the community who told a story about a giant hen whose head resided in heaven and its feet on earth. Story after story followed.

As the sun became a mere glimpse of light, I drove off with Papa John. I had just been among the poorest and most destitute people on earth, yet I had felt more connected to them than to many of my neighbors in Minnesota. The Industrial Revolution in all its glory stripped us of this gentle agricultural communal way of life. In many ways we should be grateful for that, but at what sacrifice? At the end of the day, people are people who need people. Modern sedentariness has predicated an era of disconnected loneliness. That art of storytelling is dying too—soon the stories will hide in unread books. I hate to admit it, but I have never told my children the Cry-a-lot, Moan-a-lot and Laugh-a-lot stories.

How does on-demand modernity capture the essence of this way of life? Not only has the landscape in which we live changed, so too has the speed at which business is conducted. In agricultural practice, nature sets the pace of living. The farm day is driven by sunrise and sunset. The seasons of growth, harvest and rest drive the year. Originally agriculture followed a seven-year cycle, where a field was farmed for six years and allowed to go fallow for the seventh. This seven-year cycle was repeated through generations. Agriculture follows the pace of nature and includes both growth and decay. Modernity is the immediacy of "now." It is old-fashioned to be slow and natural; it is modern to be fast and concrete.

3. Beijing, China

China has seen one of the fastest expansions of childhood obesity and chronic disease, such as diabetes, in the developing world; today one in two children in Beijing have obesity.[1] I was invited to Beijing just before the 2008 Olympics to discuss this new phenomenon. I spoke in the Great Hall of the People's Republic.

After my lecture, I was presented with two 500-year-old silver Chinese necklaces. The necklaces were similar: the neckbands were about an inch thick, and attached to each neckband was a silver box the size of a cigarette pack. The box contained a cavity in which a letter was placed. An official would write a letter, the letter would be placed inside of the box, and the box would be sealed and soldered around the neck of the courier. The courier would then carry this letter sometimes hundreds of miles to the recipient. The time between writing and reading could be weeks. Contrast this with a text message.

Of course, the immediacy of text messages is convenient, but consider for a second the quality of what is written. The handwritten letter was carried by neck in the silver necklace over hundreds of miles and would have been written in calligraphy using handmade inks painted on handmade papers. The words were carefully selected and intricately scribed.

SLOW TO QUICK: HOW NATURAL AGRICULTURALISTS BECAME CONCRETE MATERIALISTS

The shift of the last 200 years can be summarized as slow to quick. How bizarre it is that while the world became fast, we stopped moving?

How did all of this occur without us noticing? We did not notice because these changes occurred over several generations. Just as my children will never know a world without cell phones, I will never comprehend a world without cars. Neither my peers nor I have any idea what it is to live an agricultural life.

THE RISE OF CHAIRDOM

As the Industrial Revolution gathered steam, people moved to the cities and began to work in factories. In 1860, Dr. Edward Smith was commissioned by the British government to study the health consequences of the Industrial Revolution. Smith, an economist, charted the urban congestion, poverty and poor nutrition of the new modern industrial society. He went into factories and from a crow's nest in the roof spent weeks observing how people functioned in these new industrial environments that were so very different from the fields from which they had come. His report, delivered to the British Parliament, was called "On the Nourishment of the Distressed Operatives."[2]

Smith reported that humans working in factories sat for a great deal of time and did not seem as active as those who still followed agricultural lifestyles. He viewed the slowing of people in these early factories—he measured their average walking speed to be 1.1 mph—as one of the distressing symptoms of industrialization. He foresaw that this new sedentary way of life, while economically productive, was detrimental health-wise. If only we had listened to him.

As the Industrial Revolution took hold, people flooded to factories, factories filled cities and urban centers grew fast. In 1860, an automobile was unheard of; people on average walked an hour to work each way or used horse-based transportation. But in 1885, the gasoline-fueled combustion engine was developed and ultimately became the modern car.

In the United States in 1895, only 300 cars were produced, rising to 4,000 cars in 1899. In 1908, Henry Ford recognized how to put together complex machines on a conveyor belt and developed his Model T automobile. From then onward, the notion of ordinary people owning cars became a reality. At the same time that Ford was inventing a machine that would end the need to walk to work, he was also developing the system by which people would not need to move at all while working. In 1930, 5 million cars were produced for the US market; ten years later, that number had grown sixfold. The car was here to stay.

The newly styled conveyor-belt factories inspired more automated offices. Offices were redesigned in order to maximize the hours that people spent seated at a desk. It was believed that by minimizing the time office workers spent away from their desks, productivity would increase. From this desire to improve efficiency (and thus profit), a widespread endeavor evolved to keep people seated at their desks.

Several changes occurred in the offices of the 1930s and 1940s, the most important being our archenemy: the desk chair. Rigid wooden and metal chairs were out; office chairs became flexible and more comfortable. They were specifically designed to keep clerical workers at work. Casters were added to some office chairs so that workers could scoot around the office without getting up. As part of the marketing of office chairs, it was realized that there needed to be a hierarchy, whereby the softest and most comfortable chair was assigned to the most successful person in the office—the boss.

Other innovations occurred as well, to help people to stay at their desks for as long as possible. The intercom, for instance, allowed a secretary to contact the boss, and vice versa, without either moving from their desk. Then the Dictaphone's popularity emerged whereby instead of a secretary physically taking dictation, a boss could dictate into a voice recorder. The recording was then dispatched to a typing pool, where sedentary typists transcribed the recorded materials. Typists, apart from a half-hour lunch break, would be confined to their typewriter for a full workday. Data management started to become mechanized. Early adding machines, for example, were too heavy to carry, so users had to remain at their desks—sentenced to their chairs. When users of these chair-promoting products began to develop physical problems, the new science of ergonomics was born.

Ergonomic practitioners found that the new breed of seated office and factory workers were developing back and eye strain, neck cramps and wrist problems. And so these new scientists started to adjust chairs, tables and conveyor belts to help seated workers sit without as much pain.

By the 1950s mass-produced and affordable cars were on the market, and people stopped walking to work. It is said that Los Angeles was deliberately built to embrace the new car industry. The city was designed so that the only effective way of getting around was by car. Also, by the 1950s people had started to leave the cities and live in suburbs, which *obligated* them to drive to work and for pleasure. As chair mania gripped the developed world, so too did fast food. Ironic: slow bodies/fast food. But the human body had not received its final insult. Enter the desktop computer.

The first desktop computers began to appear in the 1970s. Macintosh computers appeared in the mid-1980s. Over the next few decades, half of the people in developed countries would come to sit and work behind a computer screen. The desktop computer shackled millions to their chairs. Once the computer arrived, insult after insult occurred: Accounts were no longer hand tallied, documents were not typed. Then came the final nail in the coffin: email.

Enter a modern American office today and before you is a sea of cubicles. Fingers tap plastic keys; the office buzz is sedate sedentariness.

The home has changed too. An average person can use up to 70 labor-saving devices before he or she gets to work; examples include coffee makers, electric razors, alarm clocks, heaters, coolers, email and drive-through breakfasts. Our daily lives are run by tools of convenience, each one of which serves to render us legless and inactive.

Many children cannot remember what it is to grind coffee by hand, wash clothes on a washboard, walk to school or work, walk to a library to get a book, buy a record, wind up an alarm clock, carry coal for home heat or wood for the stove. In the name of efficiency, we've gotten legless.

THE CALORIE COST OF URBANIZATION: DATA FROM JAMAICA

A decade ago, I was in my office when I received a phone call to ask if I'd meet a visiting scientist from the West Indies. An hour later, I shook the hand of Professor Terrence Forrester. Terrence is six foot four, as handsome as Denzel Washington, with a voice so musical that every sentence sounds as if it is a lullaby.

Professor Forrester was already a senior leader at the University of West Indies in Kingston. He asked if he could come to my laboratory for a year, as he was trying to understand a new health catastrophe he was seeing in Jamaica: rocketing rates of obesity and diabetes. The agricultural industry was collapsing, and people were relocating to Kingston, the capital. He had noticed an explosion in diabetes rates in Kingstonites, associated with their growing waistlines. From the land of the world's greatest sprinters, Terrence hypothesized, "People are not meant to be stuffed in cities and crammed in chairs behind tiny desks." He wanted to understand what was happening to the human body as people migrated from agriculture into the city.

I agreed to urgently visit Jamaica (yes, I know—your heart bleeds for me) with Terrence. I would at last be able to examine the natural amount of walking and sitting a rural human might do. How much sitting results from the transition from agriculture to city? How much walking have humans sacrificed with modernization?

Terrence and I arrived in Kingston midafternoon, and we were met by a driver from the university. We slowly crossed Kingston in bumper-to-bumper traffic. Hordes of children in blue uniforms were walking home. I asked the driver where these children lived. He explained that they lived in villages two hours' walk away. I thought how, in the United States, children stood on street corners feet from their homes, waiting to be collected by a school bus that would drive them to school.

The following morning, we headed to the agricultural region—a banana plantation four hours away. I was introduced to the plantation workers and the villagers. All exhibited a sense of happiness, tainted by anxiety. Theirs was a simple way of life but a precarious one at the mercy of hurricanes. I observed the different tasks on the plantation. For instance, some women stood all day over long trays of bananas floating in water and hand sifted the bananas for blemishes, casting aside the bruised ones. I met workers who laid paths in the mud to show which banana clusters would be cut on any given day. Most interesting and most terrifying, however, were the banana cutters.

Bananas grow in torso-sized clusters that hang off five-foot plants. Each cluster contains about 15 rows (called "hands") of bananas; each row comprises about 20 fruit, and so a whole cluster contains about 300 bananas. A carrier grabs a hanging cluster and places it just above his back. Then the cutter swipes a machete at the root of the cluster so that it falls onto the carrier's back. The carrier then loads the cluster onto the water-filled trays for sorting. I watched and took notes.

The plantation manager suddenly asked if I would like to try to cut a torso-sized banana cluster. Instantly and without thinking (a fault of mine), I agreed. The carrier grabbed a cluster and brought it down just above his back. I was handed a machete and told "One quick cut." I swiped the machete. It sliced through the root of the cluster as if it were sun-softened butter, with the blade coming within a finger's breadth of the carrier's head.

Thereafter Terrence's team recruited people working on the plantation and in the villages. The data would help us understand the activity levels of people living in agricultural regions. All sorts of people joined in. We had dancers, hairdressers, field workers and banana carriers, sorters and cutters. Because the activity measurement equipment contained a mass of wires, one of our participants was arrested for being a potential terrorist. We did not include the day he spent in prison as part of our data collection, but the man completed the studies anyway.

When we compared the activity levels of these agricultural dwellers to urbanites living in inner-city Kingston, what we found blew our minds.

People living in the agricultural community, regardless of whether they were dancers or banana workers, sat only half as much as their peers living in urban Kingston. On any given day, agricultural workers sat for only three hours. Once a person moved to Kingston, sitting time doubled and walking time halved. Interestingly, urbanites in Kingston sat just as much as thin urbanites living in North America. Agricultural life made people move; modern urban life made people sit. The differences were so large that it staggered us—when you live in an urban setting, even if you are lean, you move *half* as much as people living in agricultural regions. The decline in calorie burn with urbanization could entirely explain the obesity epidemic worldwide.

The first time I went to Beijing about ten years ago, throngs of bicycles went down W Changan Avenue toward the government buildings and Tiananmen Square. On the side of the road were men and women with toolboxes and repair kits. Their full-time jobs were to service the punctures and breakdowns of the thousands of bicycles running through the capital city. When I returned to Beijing a few years ago, these repairmen and women had vanished. Now that W Changan Avenue is thronged with cars, there are few bicycles and many growing bellies. The government in China is currently planning to spend $6 trillion on new city infrastructure and to urbanize 400 million agricultural dwellers. This degree of change in China mirrors Britain and the United States at the start of the Industrial Revolution. History repeats itself; unless China awakens, its obesity epidemic will make the US and European statistics look like pocket change. It may even be too late; one in two children in Beijing already have obesity, and obesity rates are accelerating faster in China than they ever did in the United States.

Studies now support the conjecture that the transition from rural to urban living precipitated chair domination.[3] In 1900, about 90 percent of the world's population was rural; a century later, more than half of the world's population lives in cities.

Since the Industrial Revolution, the inhabited world has become a network of concrete metropolises. Country by country and city by city, we have taken to our chairs at work, by car and at play. But at what cost? The human being was never designed to sit all day.

QUIZ

Have you been mechanized? How many of these 20 things can be done using machines?

1. Get to work
2. Bake bread
3. Mix a drink
4. Compact trash
5. Grind coffee
6. Wake up
7. Buy clothes
8. Heat water
9. Write a love letter
10. Listen to a story
11. Create art or music
12. Express anguish
13. Shop for fresh vegetables
14. Cool your house
15. Cut down a tree
16. Breathe
17. Have a heartbeat

18. Be intimate with your partner
19. Get a massage
20. Have a baby

The answer is *all* of them. Some machines are lifesavers; others are tools of sedentariness. It is not machines that kill people; it is how we use them.

PART II

THE CHAIRMAN'S CURSE

5

THE CHAIR-CURSED BODY

HOW DO CHAIRS KILL?

Humans were not designed to sit. Being crammed into a chair all day long is as unnatural as eating all day long. It seemed logical that sitting would be associated with illness, but I needed to prove it. To topple The Chairman, Professor Smallbrain and Dr. Micromind, I needed help—I need the Cricketers' Brain Trust.

The Cricketers' Brain Trust is one of the world's leading scientific groups in diabetes research. Its members, Yogish Kudva, Andy Basu, Chinmay Manohar and their boss, Rita Basu, work at Mayo Clinic.

Yogish, or Dr. Brain, is a living encyclopedia on diabetes and pretty much everything else. He remembers facts, names and scientific papers, often from decades before. If Wikipedia ever goes bust, Yogish can replace it. Andy, intense, mustached and penetrating, is the Hercule Poirot of treating adult-type diabetes. Chinmay is a young technological genius. In a few hours, he can throw together a few microchips and create a working technology. In meetings he might say barely eight words, but each one is patentable. Finally, there is Rita, who controls "the boys" with the power of a Roman charioteer and the intellect of Ruth Bader Ginsburg.

The members of the Cricketers' Brain Trust know diabetes. Hypothesizing that the chair might be partially to blame for an epidemic of diabetes[1] running riot across the developed world, they wanted to perform experiments to prove their idea. So they called a meeting.

Yogish began. He explained that after a meal, a person's blood sugar climbs to mountainous levels. It peaks after about 60 minutes and then declines for the next few hours. The body handles this spike in blood sugar in part by having the body make more insulin, which pushes the sugar into the "stand and walk" muscles of the thighs, buttocks and trunk. Yogish reeled off the names of genes that function in the individual muscle cells to handle the extra insulin and blood sugar. Most had names that are easily forgotten—GLUT4, FABP1 and so on. He saw me glazing over and said, "Jim, look, it's simple! When you eat a meal, your blood sugar shoots up, your pancreas pushes out insulin and the insulin drives the meal's sugar into the muscle."

Andy could see I was still lost. He stroked his mustache and summarized: "Basically, when you eat, the pancreas squirts out insulin, so that the muscles and other vital organs get the glucose they need. Any sugar left over gets converted into fat."

Chinmay smiled, adding, "That's what we think is wrong with sitting; if you sit, you do not use your meal sugar and so you get diabetes."

Yogish joined in, explaining that the body is designed to activate dozens of systems (he started to list them) so that when you eat the food, fuel is made available to the individual muscle cells and organs that need it. This fuel-delivery system, he explained, is designed to allow the body to be continuously active after eating.

I thought back to when I worked in Jamaica and the Ivory Coast, where workers ate breakfast at dawn and labored all morning in the fields. They then took a break for lunch and afterward returned to manual work. It made sense—the food you eat needs to be delivered to the muscle to be used for active work. If you spend the afternoon sitting in front of your computer, the fuel is unused and so ends up as fat.

Andy said what I was thinking: "The trouble is, Jim, nowadays everyone eats but no one physically works their body afterward."

Yogish bumped the table excitedly. His voice was getting louder. "Jim, all of the cells and molecular mechanisms are built on the premise that the body moves all the time because we work physically. That's the whole problem; today we eat three meals, sit all day and are not physical at all. The cellular engines were *never* built to sit. When we sit all the day, the surplus fuel is washing around the bloodstream like a massive oil slick in the ocean."

Chinmay added, "That's why we think a third of the population has elevated blood sugar, called prediabetes, and one in ten adults actually has diabetes." I waited for him to say something else, but he was silent.

Andy spoke. "If you sit all day long and all of the muscle engines are idle, and the surplus blood sugar fills the bloodstream, what do you think happens next?" He paused. "Diabetes."

Yogish added passionately, "The American Diabetes Association defines prediabetes as a blood sugar above 100 and below 126 milligrams per deciliter. Seventy-nine million Americans have prediabetes. Two-thirds of people with prediabetes go on to develop full-blown diabetes within ten years." He paused. "Diabetes is an elevated blood sugar equal [to] or above 126 and 26 million people have diabetes, mostly adult-type diabetes. Every year there are 2 million new cases of diabetes diagnosed. For every two people diagnosed with diabetes, there is someone else who has it but does not know. The annual cost of diabetes is $6,700 per person."[2]

The more I thought about the cause of diabetes, the more I understood why the Cricketers' Brain Trust wanted to study sitting. Because most of us are sedentary all day, our blood sugar rises hugely after each meal. Our sedentary muscle cells never use the sugar we consume; instead, it swirls around the bloodstream. The body tries to fight this by making more insulin to suppress the elevated blood sugar. But then, after constant overexposure to high levels of insulin, the body becomes insensitive to it. The mixture of high blood sugar and high blood insulin is diabetes. The huge spikes in blood glucose after each meal would not occur if people moved after they ate, just as we're designed to do.

Rita stepped in. "We need to do some studies, to get data," she said. We all looked to her. Andy brushed his mustache. "It would be fascinating," he suggested, "to meticulously measure the mountainous climbs of blood sugar after each meal and then see what happens if somebody walks after their meal like they used to do." Yogish interjected, "We could perform complex mathematics to examine whether walking after a meal can lower the elevations of blood glucose and potentially prevent diabetes. The trouble is," he concluded, "we need a technology that can measure blood sugar and nonexercise-NEAT activity every second before and after a meal." All eyes fell on Chinmay. He smiled. "We can do that."

A year later, the studies were published.[3] Blood sugar and NEAT movements were measured continuously every second before and after volunteers consumed meals. The data were irrefutable and startling. If people sit after a meal, their blood sugar peaks like a mountain for about two hours. If, however, people take a 15-minute walk at 1 mph after a meal, the mountains become safe, gentle, rolling hills. With a 1-mph walk after a meal, blood sugar peaks are *halved*. Looking at the data was life changing. People can lower their high blood sugar after a meal simply by taking a short walk after they eat. The day I saw the data was the day I changed. Whether it's breakfast, lunch or dinner—after every meal, I take a short NEAT walk, usually for 15 minutes. The Cricketers' Brain Trust had discovered why the chair causes diabetes.

Food is fuel. We consume food to propel the body. If you sit instead, mountain-high blood sugar values result. With chair addiction on the rise, no wonder diabetes rates are predicted to double.

THE AUSTRALIANS COME TO TOWN

Just as the Cricketers' Brain Trust was publishing its data in 2012, I went to a meeting hosted by a furniture company called Ergotron. Ergotron was getting into the NEAT business, building standing desks. It had convened an international panel to learn more about the sitting disease. I paced at the back of the room and listened to the lectures; my presentation was not until the end of the day.

Throughout the day, I noticed a young sandy-haired man watching me. At the afternoon coffee break, he tapped me on the shoulder. "I'm giving the presentation after yours," he said. Professor David Duncan was from the Baker IDI Heart and Diabetes Institute in Australia. His team had addressed the issue of diabetes and sedentariness in a different way. It had taken a group of people who are normally active and imposed a chair sentence on them. The people were made to sit for days on end. The team discovered that the more these people sat, the worse their blood sugars became. However, intermittently moving could dramatically improve blood sugar values. His conclusion was the same as that of the Cricketers' Brain Trust: Sitting causes diabetes. David said, "Create opportunities within your waking hours to limit sitting time." He went on to explain that for every hour you sit watching television or listening to a lecture, your life expectancy decreases by 22 minutes.[4] By the time his lecture finished, the entire audience was slowly pacing up and down the room.[5]

The plot was about to get thicker. Enter Professor Mark Hamilton, a physiologist from Louisiana who looks more like a choirboy. Although he is a superb scientist, what intrigues me about Mark is his fervor. He had conducted some unusual experiments. In one he'd taken rats and raised their hind legs in a harness. These animals existed quite happily without having to carry most of their own weight. It was an animal model of sedentary living. He discovered that these rats were prone to very high levels of triglycerides, one of the components of the cholesterol system. These high triglycerides were associated with the rats' sluggishness, hardening of the arteries and diabetes.[6] Mark also measured thousands of genes from their muscles—sedentariness was associated with multiple gene changes in the muscle cells (the same ones that Yogish pointed out contributed to diabetes). The evidence was accumulating: Fundamental changes in biology occur if you sit for too long.

Mark later conducted studies in humans rather similar to the Australian group. He would bring people into his research center and make them sit all day long. Repeatedly sampling their blood, he examined what happened to the cholesterol system if you force a person to become chairbound. The data were astounding. Even in people with well-controlled cholesterol, he saw values of triglycerides rise so high as to be associated with cardiovascular disease.[7] At the same time, data were coming in from epidemiologists from around the world. For example, Japanese scientists found that the less you walk, the worse your cholesterol panel.[8] Swedish scientists showed that the more you sit, the progressively greater your risk of a heart attack.[9] Dutch scientists found that sedentariness was associated with stiffening arteries.[10] German scientists demonstrated that excessive sitting softens the skeleton.[11] The evidence base was deepening. One study from Sydney looked at 22,497 Australian adults. People who sat 11 hours or more per day had a 40 percent greater risk of premature death than people who sat for four hours or less. Sitting accounted for 7 percent of all premature deaths.[12] It was clear that the chair sentence extends beyond obesity; if you sit too long, diabetes, osteoporosis, heart disease and early death follow.

Added to diabetes, obesity and heart disease came new culprits of the chair sentence. Cancers of the breast, colon, lung and endometrium,[13] depression, hypertension, back pain and poor sleep quality were associated with prolonged sitting. And it's not subtle—for example, regardless of a woman's body weight, strolling for an hour a day reduces breast cancer risk by 14 percent, compared with being sedentary.[14]

A few years ago, I heard Mark Hamilton lecture in Miami; he showed the classic image of the Marlboro Cowboy astride his horse. Sitting is more dangerous than smoking, he explained. Professor Steven Blair was also at this meeting. One of the masters of the exercise revolution, he explained that 18 percent of the population smokes and smokers get lung cancer, cardiovascular disease and asthma; nonsmokers, 82 percent of the population, don't get smoking illnesses. Professor Blair went on to explain that more than three-quarters of Americans sit all day long. Therefore, the total population risks associated with sitting, when you add them all up, are far greater than the risks associated with smoking. I had been quoted in the press as saying, "Sitting is the new smoking." I was wrong; if you look at America as a whole, sitting is *worse* than smoking!

You might have thought that going to the gym protects you from lethal sitting. If you are one of the 15 percent of Americans who belongs to a gym, I have something eye-opening to tell you. Going to the gym, even several times a week, does not reverse the harmful effects of prolonged sitting. Dr. Emma Wilmot at the University of Leicester explained. "People convince themselves they are living a healthy lifestyle, doing their 30 minutes of exercise a day. But they need to think about the other 23.5 hours."[15] People who go to the gym do *not* reverse the health impact of prolonged sitting.[16] Even if you go to the gym, excessive sitting kills.

Lastly, it does not matter what age you are; chair-sentenced elderly are less able to manage the tasks of daily living compared to more active peers.[17]

Although it is a good sound bite—"Sitting is the new smoking"—the concept is important. Knowledge about sitting disease has grown exponentially with about 10,000 scientific publications in the last 15 years. Leading experts agree that sitting actually causes more ill health than smoking. The chair sentence affects people of all ages, both sexes and from multiple countries. The ill effects of sitting, the chair disease, are a shopping list of misery.

Think of the size of the anti-smoking lobby, the campaigns against smoking, the funds invested in stop-smoking programs and the catalogs of anti-smoking legislation. Where is the anti-chair lobby and stand-not-sit legislation? Up until now, there has not been a movement to reverse the chair sentence, although government bodies are beginning to hear the call; Australia, Europe, the United States and Canada all in the last few years formally recognized the harm of prolonged sitting.[18]

Get up! You can prevent prediabetes from becoming diabetes and prehypertension from becoming hypertension. Sitters die sooner—for every hour you sit, two hours of life walk away!

QUIZ

Here is the ABC of illnesses associated with excessive sitting. Without looking ahead at the question that follows, please read through this list with care. When you are done, read the question.

HARMFUL EFFECTS OF SITTING

A—Arthritis

B—Blood pressure, back pain

C—Cancer, cholesterol problems

D—Diabetes, dementia

E—Emphysema, exacerbation of asthma

F—Fat gain

G—Gestational diabetes

H—Heart attack

I—Immobility, isolation, infertility, impaired glucose metabolism

J—Joint aches

K—Kyphosis of back, kidney problems

L—Loneliness, leg swelling

M—Moodiness, muscle ache

N—Nutricide (death caused by poor nutrition), nerve entrapment (e.g., carpal tunnel)

O—Obesity, obstructive sleep apnea, osteoporosis

P—Poor productivity, Potts disease

Q—Quality of life

R—Relationship problems

S—Stigmatization, sedentary minds, swollen ankles, sexual dysfunction

T—Trapped feeling, tendonitis

U—Underachiever, unhappiness

V—Varicose veins

W—Wasted opportunities

X—X-rated angst and impaired performance

Y—Yearning for something better

Z—Zest

Here's the question: You have just read through a list of the ills associated with sitting. Are you still sitting down?

6

THE CHAIR-CURSED MIND

STRESS, STRESS! THIS STRESS IS KILLING ME!

The most highly stressed period of my life was when I got divorced. My ex-wife and two children went back to the United Kingdom, leaving me in Minnesota. The day they left was one of the saddest in my life.

I remember going to the parking lot at Minneapolis Airport and getting in my car. The lot was dimly lit. From habit, I glanced in the rearview mirror at the pair of car seats. I could still hear the voices of my girls in the silence. I could smell them. It was cold and the car seats were empty. I started the engine, and the silence became an engine drone.

I did not drive away but just sat in the silence, the silence of "missing."

That night I went back to my two-bedroom, newly-divorced-man rental. The next day I spoke with my two daughters, now 4,000 miles away. Their telephone sounds and distant words did not fill the void I felt. That void never goes away; you just move it to somewhere else in your head.

A week later, I was going through the Mayo hospital cafeteria line and pushed my tray past the drink counter; I saw cartons of chocolate milk. Often on Sundays my eldest daughter came to work with me. "Drink the chocolate milk," I would bargain with her. That lunchtime, I saw the chocolate milk, looked down and she wasn't there. I was struck still.

I don't know how I got back home. I went to their room—left as though they were about to visit—and started to cry. I cried until I fell asleep and woke up on the floor between their empty beds; my pager was going off. I had a patient to see.

In the depression that followed, everything white was gray and every shadow a cavern. People were around, friends called to help, but I stopped hearing them. The TV calmed me and microwave pizza warmed me. I stopped fencing, something I had done twice a week. Work became a distraction. I would listen to patients with heightened interest and ask them about how they felt. Many of my patients with obesity live daily with pain, not only from their medical ailments, but from discrimination, stigmatization and self-reproach; my sense of personal pain was so great that I somehow felt closer to the needs of my patients.

When I wasn't with patients, I was in the lab peering at data as if hidden truths would answer my problems. Work became a safe place; patients in the morning, the lab in the afternoon and sometimes all night. The treadmill desk was in my office—still. I never switched it on.

I knew that I was a rubbish father because my children were so far away. I knew that they wanted me almost as much as I wanted them, so I began monthly treks to London. I would live for those weekends, be happy and then die again.

I gained weight. As I sat more, my sadness worsened. The sadder I became, the more I ate. As work became my sole salvation, I started to view my chair as my safe place. In my clinic room, my doctor's chair became my place for curing people—for making other people feel better. My lab chair became my place for discovering new universes—as if I could escape there. My home chair became my place to eat, watch TV, study for my board exams and sleep. From one chair to the next, my sadness grew, and my waistband expanded. Then I discovered banana liqueur. I love the taste of banana; my record was half a bottle in one night. I had sunk as low as I could let myself. If living is a journey, I had lost sight of the destination.

The first time I made an appointment to see a psychiatrist, I canceled it. The second time, I sat in the waiting room for 30 minutes and then left. The third time, I made it from the waiting room's chair to the patient's chair.

"Why are you here?" the psychiatrist asked. Dr. K was my age. Her gaze was firm, like that of a car mechanic who actually knows what that strange whirring is under the passenger seat. "You can tell me," she said. "I am a rubbish dad," I replied.

SAD SITTING

My depression became like a heavy blanket and kept me down in my chair. I had given up fencing, eating right, going to museums. I stopped going to theaters and concerts. I felt ashamed to go to professional dinners; I'd be the only one without a spouse—they all knew. I could not play with my kids because they were not there. I did not impose this chair sentence on myself; it was a symptom of my despair. I was down, done, fat and out.

This cycle of what I call "sad sitting" is commonplace. Getting up—whatever it takes—is part of the cure. Walking regularly—each day, even for just half an hour—is used for prevention and as part of the treatment for depression.[1] People with depression have a symptom called anhedonia, which refers to the lack of interest in *anything*. The chair is the inevitable home of the sad. The chair is where people who are sad end up. I did. One in five Americans develops depression at some time in her life. The chair becomes the depressive's sanctuary.

On my fourth visit, Dr. K said, "You are either going to show me you can break this cycle or you're taking medication. I don't think you need inpatient care right now, but I'm not taking it off the table." She gave me an activity diary. I had to write down one positive thing I did *for myself* each day—work, TV and pizza did not count. That night I drove to Minneapolis to fence. The best part about fencing was that the fencers knew nothing of my family going away. I was chastised for being out of shape; the eight-year-olds were creaming me!

SAD SITTING: CAUSE *AND* EFFECT?

But there is another aspect to sad sitting, one that is more insidious. If walking helps reverse depression, can enforced sitting *cause* sadness?

What happens to the brain when we sit that might make us sad?[2] Most of the data comes from chair-sentenced rats. When you force a rat to be inactive, its muscles fire less because they are not stimulated. In people, that decrease in muscle firing may cause the parts of the brain that make you active to shrink. (The brain is like a muscle—if you don't use it, it shrinks.) The shrunken activity center of the brain sends out fewer signals to move. You move even less, the brain's activity center shrinks more and the cycle repeats itself. The brain adapts to your chair sentence. If the chair seduces a person, his muscles sense it, his brain adapts and he becomes sad and sluggish and feels depressed. People who sit adapt to sit more and become sadder.

Consider what happens when you break the sit-sad cycle and take a vacation; you get more sleep, hopefully more sex, perhaps eat more, but also often become more active. A vacation is a temporary escape from the chair sentence. Science backs this up: An active body begets an active brain. When people who have been sedentary walk more, they feel better, brighter, more energized and smarter. It stands to reason that moving more is linked in the brain's circuitry to feeling happier. Sad sitting can be reversed, but as I discovered, you have to get up to break the cycle.

THE STRESS EFFECT

Over the years, the Mayo NEAT team has conducted chair-release consultancies in countless corporations. The commonest complaint we hear isn't about pay or hours but *stress*. Stress comes in many forms, from balancing work and kids, job security and challenging work relationships (e.g., with a terrible boss).

There is a tendency to believe that stress is all bad. This is not so.[3] Stress is a natural human response. If you are not stressed out by a saber-toothed tiger charging at you, you become cat food! What is wrong with modern living is how we deal with stressors. We do not routinely get up and run in response to stress; we sit and eat! Stress is one of the most common reasons clients explain excess eating, although the actual stressors vary: rushing, "pressure" and loneliness are frequent examples.[4]

When researchers examined data from 76 studies, they found that some types of work stress are good; for instance, if you have a presentation due tomorrow and you have the right skills to pull it off, the stress of the deadline will actually help you improve your presentation.[5] Negative stress, however, is more common. For instance, if your office is chaotic *and* you are chasing 30 tasks simultaneously *and* your kids need soccer cleats *and* you have to be at soccer practice in a few hours, adding three more tasks (increasing the chaos) induces negative stress, and everything gets done less well. You may recognize this scenario as modern multitasking.

Chronic unrelenting negative stress is like pounding a hammer against a bathtub; eventually the tub will crack. Most often people internalize chronic stress by drinking, eating or self-medicating before it is redirected into anger or negative behaviors, such as violence or high-risk sexual behaviors.

Stress at the brain level is associated with a cascade of stress hormones.[6] High stress influences the melanocortin system. This system, housed in the hypothalamus and the brain stem, is linked to the pituitary gland at the base of the brain, which produces a hormone called corticotropin. Corticotropin leaves the brain, enters the blood stream and heads to the adrenal glands, just above the kidneys, to produce the stress hormone, cortisol.

The hypothalamus-pituitary-corticotropin-cortisol cascade is a stress system common to a number of animals.[7] During periods of long-term stress, cortisol levels increase. Among early humans, this was valuable; natural stressors were life threatening, so the body developed a response system. The body, however, was never designed for the unrelenting stress of an awful boss, getting kids to gymnastics and soccer, paying rent and keeping a third job while sitting all day. We know from patients who have high cortisol levels—for instance, those with Cushing's disease (caused by a tumor that makes excess cortisol)—that high cortisol levels can do significant harm to the mind and body.

EXCESS CORTISOL LEADS TO STRESSED-OUT BODIES

In medical school, my first professor in endocrinology came from the north of England. He was brash and brilliant, not a man who held back comment or criticism nor feared controversy. My first patient with Cushing's disease had increased his eating and gained 40 pounds. His blood pressure was terrible, and his bone scan showed soft bones. I reported all of these facts to the professor. The professor barked, "But how does the patient *feel?*" The doctor towered over me by a foot. I looked at his shoes and shrugged. We went to see the patient together. With patients, the harsh giant was kindness personified. He held the man's hand and asked, "So how have you been doing?" The patient was from a tough part of London, but a tear rolled down his cheek. "That bad," said my professor, and looked at me. He summarized, "You see, Levine, too much cortisol makes patients fat and frumpy."

This is a vicious cycle: The more stress you have, the more cortisol your body releases.[8] As a result of the excess cortisol, you eat more (the melanocortin system, described above, directly impacts appetite), feel sadder ("frumpy"), gain weight and sit. The cortisol system numbs the muscles' responses to "move-it" stimuli, making it more likely that you'll sit in the first place.[9] Because oftentimes, negative stress is unrelenting, you then eat even more, gain even more weight and your vulnerability to further stress-related fat gain is even greater. To add salt to the wound, gaining weight is itself stressful; people with obesity are discriminated against and feel ostracized, which pumps up stress levels and cortisol even further.[10] As a result of this vicious cycle, you get more stressed and the cortisol-sit-sadness-cycle perpetuates. After a while, diabetes and high blood pressure occur and add to the burden.

The population-wide stress experiment is called the modern office. The chair sentence prevents your stress from ever being cured: It prevents the cortisol cycle from ever being broken. The modern office stops you from getting up. How many hundreds of office clients with obesity have told me that they eat under stress? Perhaps if they had not been chair sentenced, they would not have stress-eaten and developed obesity in the first place.

If you see a saber-toothed tiger charging toward you, you don't fire off an email, you get up and run! If life is stressing you out, break the cortisol cycle and get up!

THE SLEEP PARADOX

When I first entered residency, the call schedule was one night in three. Every third night, instead of going home at 5 p.m., I worked through the night and then the next day. The on-call room and on-call lounge were stocked with free sandwiches and soda—a junior doctor's dream.

At night, I avoided Diet Coke because of the caffeine and instead drank lemonade. When admissions from the ER slowed down, I would try to nap but could never sleep. At 3 a.m. I would raid the free sandwiches, have free breakfast at 8 a.m. and then have lunch and a snack. After the 40-hour stretch, I would get home exhausted, collapse into a chair, eat and then sleep. Every third night was the same.

That is what sleep deprivation does to you. Because you are up for longer, you eat more, but you do *not* move more. If you are sleep deprived, you are exhausted, move less and sit more. Sleep deprivation causes obesity—more food, more chair!

To better understand the impact of sleep on NEAT and sitting, I began working with Virend Somers, the Einstein of the sleep world. Dr. Somers had many years' experience not only in measuring how people sleep but also the effects of experimental sleep deprivation. Shelly McCrady-Spitzer, from my lab, is the Madame Curie of the NEAT world; she began to organize a collaboration between Somers's lab and ours. Together, we conducted a unique sleep deprivation study. We recruited healthy people who were willing to be sleep deprived for 21 consecutive days for the good of humankind.[11] Our volunteers became exhausted, and we measured their responses. The less they slept, the more they ate and the more they sat. Sleep deprivation and obesity sit beside each other on the sofa.

WHY IS SLEEP IMPORTANT?

While the human body sleeps, not only does it switch off, but it also enters a self-repair mode. Growth hormone, which is crucial for muscle and bone maintenance, is mostly released while we sleep. The proteins associated with causing dementia are cleared from the brain when people sleep. Also, sleep is necessary for optimized insulin release and diabetes prevention. More subtly, while we sleep, we dream. Sigmund Freud suggested that sleep plays a critical role in repairing the psyche. But also, neuroscientists suggest, while we sleep, a host of neurocircuits are repaired and memories are saved.[12]

Sleep is different from sitting, even though in both cases we do not move much. When we sit and stare at our computer screens, our bodies are like idling engines. The inactive muscles are understimulated and so break down. When you sit, your body's natural insulin is less effective; and so sitting is associated with elevated blood sugar and diabetes. With respect to the psyche, we get stressed while seated at work. Your manager may be as threatening as a saber-toothed tiger, but you have to *sit* through the stress, internalize it and the cortisol cycle is perpetuated. While we sit, our blood triglycerides creep up and up, and our hearts function sluggishly. Blood flow is not returned efficiently from our legs, and our ankles swell. Back pain occurs and our wrists hurt. Prolonged sitting softens the skeleton. As we continue to stay seated, our brains lull and creativity falls. Sleep is as good for us as sitting is bad.

Data suggest that daytime naps benefit the body and energize us to be more active afterward.[13] Once I had seen the results from Virend and Shelly's sleep deprivation study, I started to take afternoon naps wherever I could.

Getting good sleep is critical to energize your chair escape. Close the book and take a nap!

SIT DOWN—MIND OFF

The NEAT lab's first office experiment was in 2008 in a Minneapolis financial services company called Salo. Workers across the company got up out of their chairs and took on NEAT-active work. As people got up, their health and happiness measures improved, but most interestingly, they also felt a new sense of personal empowerment.

In one case, a woman decided that she wanted to sing at her parents' fiftieth wedding anniversary. She started to take singing lessons (practicing in the car going to and from work). Not only did she sing at the anniversary celebration, she began a new career (in her off hours) as a jazz singer. Another of our volunteers called me up one morning at 5 a.m. He couldn't restrain himself. "Dr. Levine. You'll never believe it. I walked a half-marathon yesterday at work . . . in my business suit." This same person, three months later, completed his first novel and now runs his own business that promotes active office cultures. In a third example, an office worker started a cooking club. Not your standard let's-share-recipes group; instead, she hired a professional cook and once a week invited friends to come to her house to learn to cook healthily. This behavior directly affected the workplace; cookies and cakes vanished and were replaced by the healthful snack of the week. The office went on to have cook-offs for prizes. In a fourth example, a worker invented *and built* her own desk-side workout equipment. A company saw this and commercialized it as a desk exercise kit. In a fifth example, a chocoholic climbed out of her chair and planned her own withdrawal program, which we now use in our programs around the country. (The trick is to buy really good chocolate, in smaller quantities, and savor it!) The final example is the most dramatic. One young worker had dreamed of teaching English in an underserved country. She got out of her chair, took a leave of absence and went to teach English in a remote part of China.

The most common observation I make when we roll out chair-release programs is that by getting up, as a first simple step, people start to regain personal power. It is as though by *physically* getting up, people are released from a sedentary *psychological* imprisonment that forbids self-propulsion, self-expression and self-fulfillment. It is true that as we ease people out of their chairs, they see improvements to their blood sugar levels, blood pressures and waistlines. However, the examples I just described tell a more compelling tale. When people get out of their chairs, they blossom as if they finally are free from prison. As people shed their chair shackles and get up, their creativity bursts out; they take steps toward their dreams and move their lives under their own power—step by step by step—forward. They remember the destination they'd always wanted to reach.

I challenge you. Stop for one minute and shut your eyes. How do you visualize yourself in your mind's eye? What do you want for yourself? Go on, close your eyes (unless you're driving or biking) and ask yourself those questions.

It is said that Einstein came up with $E=mc^2$ while biking across the Princeton University campus. Get out of your chair and become the person you dream of being.

STRESS TEST

Find the following words in this puzzle. You have two minutes.
Set your timer. Go!

BODY	MISERABLE
CHAIR	OUT
COMFORT	SAD
CORTISOL	SENTENCE
EATING	SITTING
FAT	STRESS
MELANOCORTIN	STRESSED

```
M  C  K  E  K  A  Y  Z  O  Z  A  W  R  Q  H
Q  E  A  L  B  C  C  S  M  T  Z  U  E  K  S
H  Z  L  B  G  O  H  X  A  E  Z  T  Y  H  K
R  C  L  A  F  N  A  F  Q  D  T  H  W  H  I
R  S  Y  R  N  D  I  A  Q  E  U  P  H  T  B
O  V  T  E  C  O  R  T  I  S  O  L  G  O  D
A  Z  Y  S  M  W  C  R  A  S  S  E  F  L  X
E  A  E  I  K  Y  C  O  U  E  I  C  H  I  B
Y  X  K  M  H  Y  B  F  R  R  T  N  K  T  Z
D  Z  W  J  C  E  D  M  D  T  T  E  D  F  Q
T  M  R  W  F  V  U  O  N  S  I  T  T  F  Y
O  H  T  E  G  I  P  C  B  X  N  N  R  O  R
T  D  E  B  Z  K  W  R  Q  N  G  E  T  R  M
K  Y  W  Y  H  W  R  D  Y  E  V  S  N  L  Y
B  N  W  W  C  K  P  V  Z  P  Q  W  O  D  J
```

Isn't it interesting how all these stress-related concepts inter-
mingle and fit together? Did you notice that "stressed" spelled
backward is "desserts"?

7

THE CHAIR-CURSED CAR

MY FIRST ENCOUNTER WITH THE MODERN URBAN JUNGLE was when I visited Los Angeles for an international scientific congress in 1987. As part of my PhD thesis, while in London, I developed a new technology for measuring human calorie burn using miniature refrigerators. These refrigerators were placed against the skin, and the power needed to keep the refrigerator cool approximated the calorie burn from the person's skin. I was excited about these miniature refrigerators, and the conference organizers agreed. I had star billing.

Marsha Morgan, my PhD mentor, was fiercely passionate about her science. I had met her halfway through medical school and said to her that I wanted to better understand how to measure how people burn calories. She smiled and said, "Then do it." "But I am not an electrical engineer and you don't have an electronics lab," I said. Dr. Morgan replied, "If you get a degree in electrical engineering, I'll get you a laboratory."

Two years later I began my PhD in electrical and computer engineering. As promised, I had my own lab at the Royal Free Hospital in London, a small, vacated examination room. The little room became my life. I moved in an oscilloscope and an array of electronic circuits and gadgets. The miniature refrigerators started to accurately measure calorie burn. Among my challenges was the fact that they required more electricity than a television despite their tiny size: They were only half an inch square. I solved that with suitcase-size power transformers.

One day I was having lunch with Marsha and my collaborator, a young dietician named Angela Madden, when we saw two fire crews sprinting past the cafeteria. When we returned to my tenth-floor lab, there was thick black smoke everywhere, and the firemen were hosing out the room; my oscilloscope (which I'd bought with my own savings) was covered in white foam. Apparently my lab had exploded. Marsha looked at the scene and then at me. "Jim," she said, "you had better do a bit more adjusting before you try it out on Olympic athletes."

I improved the miniature refrigerator system, this time with exhaustive safety features, and we tested the technology at the Olympic training station in North London. It enabled us to measure heat loss from individual muscle groups in long-distance runners. It never exploded again, and the athletes loved it. Marsha, Angela and I headed off to Los Angeles to present our findings.

Marsha was staying at the Hilton, near Rodeo Drive, Angela stayed in a Holiday Inn near the convention center and I was staying in a youth hostel. I rented a car and, using a large map (this was long before GPS existed), navigated the concrete jungle of Los Angeles, a city specifically built to *not* encourage walking. The 10,000 miles of roadways were meant to promote driving and bolster the car industry.

I found Rodeo Drive and picked up Marsha. Then we collected Angela from the Holiday Inn, and off we went to the convention center. We presented our data to an appreciative audience, and afterward I made the mistake of accepting the glass of champagne Marsha shoved in my hand. At about 10 p.m., I offered to drive the women back to their respective hotels. Heading out of the convention center, I had to follow a one-way road system, and, at the crucial moment, I took a wrong turn. Soon I was hopelessly lost. My companions were not pleased.

When a traffic light turned red, I stopped. Groups of men advanced toward the car from right and left. Marsha's hands gripped her handbag; I looked at her. Her face had hardened. From the back of the car Angela called, "Jim!" Two men had come from behind the car and were reaching toward the door handle. As if by instinct, my foot slammed on the accelerator, and we drove through the red light, ducking oncoming traffic and an orchestra of car horns. A block later, lights appeared in my rearview mirror. I was being pulled over. A policeman came up to the car and stared inside. Marsha flashed a smile. The policeman smiled back and looked at me. "What are you doing in this neighborhood?" he asked. I said, "I'm lost." He didn't even check my license or registration but said, "You should not be here, sir. I am going to drive you out of here; follow me."

I went to several more conferences with Marsha. She never asked me to drive her again.

Los Angeles is the perfect example of a modern concrete jungle. Concrete roadways connect multimillion-dollar privately secured neighborhoods to dangerous, gang-controlled districts.[1]

Several years after my first visit to LA, I was invited to lecture there by Peter Butler, a dashing Kenyan-born professor who ran a famous diabetes center. I showed up at 9 a.m. at the Keck School of Medicine, a full hour early for our meeting, to discover that he actually worked at the University of California, Los Angeles, 18 miles away. I ran to my car, sat in traffic for two hours, shared road rage with thousands of others and arrived more than an hour late. Los Angeles has the most congested streets in the United States and third-most congested, after Brussels and Antwerp, in the world.[2] The average LA driver experiences 72 hours of traffic delay per year—that's nearly two workweeks. Overall, US drivers waste 3 billion gallons of gas per year and 6 billion hours sitting in traffic.[3]

WALK IT OFF

California generates about 7 percent of US greenhouse gas emissions, which ranks it the number 12 emitter in the world.[4] Cars account for 80 percent of these emissions, and the city of Los Angeles contributes the most. Great urban centers were a vision of the Industrial Revolution. LA is one representation of this dream, having the third-largest metropolitan economy ($639 billion) in the world after Tokyo and New York.[5]

Over the last century, the number of cars in use in the world has increased to meet people's travel demands. On a global scale, a quarter of global emissions are transportation related, with cars accounting for the vast majority of these pollutants.[6] Looking at the expansion of car sales, especially in China and India, car exhaust is anticipated to grow faster than your stock portfolio.

Car pollutants aren't just carbon monoxide; they also include nitrogen oxide and volatile organic compounds. The World Health Organization estimates that 1.3 million people die prematurely each year from air pollution, with the car being the number one cause of this pollution.[7] In fact, people living close to a major roadway are likely to die from cardiovascular illness, respiratory illness and lung cancer.[8] In the same way that the desk chair and sofa are the agents of death at work and home, so too is the car seat for the times in between.

It is obvious that solving the chair sentence is not going to involve leveling Los Angeles. However, can we do things differently? Can we realistically get out of our cars and walk?

Active leg-based transportation is common in a number of European cities, such as Copenhagen and Amsterdam. Rain or shine, Amsterdam is swamped with bicycles. When I was last there, it poured continuously for three days, but still people cycled everywhere, some holding umbrellas at the same time.

Detailed analyses of the implications for transforming car-dense inner-city areas into areas with more leg-based transportation have been made. In one example, British researchers analyzed the implications of making a typical Victorian terraced inner-city street more physically active by 2030.[9] At the start of the study, the street was crowded with parked cars, and people on the sidewalks looked cramped. In the most advanced scenario, the road was essentially carless and people walked and cycled at ease. No construction was necessary. With this transformation, carbon dioxide emissions would decline by more than 80 percent. Although these changes would result in people walking and/or bicycling 26 minutes extra per day, their daily commute was extended only by 7 minutes. The change in car use in this scenario could decrease heart disease, diabetes and dementia by 15 percent each.

The potential health benefits for reversing car-seat sedentariness are similar for the United States. For San Francisco in 2013, the average person's travel time by foot was 4 minutes per day. In an active San Francisco leg-based travel scenario, average daily foot and bicycle commutes would increase by 18 minutes. Overall, the health benefits for the extra 18 daily minutes of walking/ bicycling are staggering; there would be a potential 13 percent reduction in premature deaths. The greatest improvements would be in decreased heart disease, diabetes, stroke, dementia, depression, cancer and road traffic accidents. For San Francisco, this translates to 2,404 avoided premature deaths per year.[10] This degree of improved health would rank among the greatest health advances in modern history. In San Francisco alone, healthcare cost savings would amount to $34 billion/year, and the profitability of neighborhood retail shops would improve.[11] Leg-based city travel is both healthful and profitable and does not add substantially to commute times.

A few years ago, I became director of Obesity Solutions at Mayo Clinic Arizona and Arizona State University (ASU). I relocated from Rochester, Minnesota, to Phoenix. Recently I went to my office in downtown Phoenix for a meeting, to the ASU campus at Tempe to teach and then to northeast Scottsdale for an administrative meeting at Mayo. After my meeting, I drove to an evening seminar in downtown Scottsdale. In total, I spent three hours in the car, traveled 40 miles, used two gallons of gas, thumped the steering wheel several times at dreadful drivers, ate lunch, spoke on the phone (hands-free) and screamed once. When I look back on the day, I could have bicycled from my home to the university at Tempe (a 30-minute ride each way) and met my other obligations on a video link or by phone.

Redesigning environments—whether they are transportation systems, offices or schools—can influence people's behavior, *but* the greatest influence on a person's behavior is the person!

CAR QUIZ

Which of the following things have you done in a car in the last month?

Eaten: 1 point

Shaved: 1 point

Talked on your cell phone as you drive: 2 points

Text messaged while driving: 3 points

Knitted: 2 points

Applied makeup: 2 points

Thumped the steering wheel: 2 points

Watched movies or TV: 2 points

Used apps: 3 points

Conducted remote robotic surgery: 3 points

Played a video game: 3 points

Folded laundry: 3 points

Shopped online: 4 points

Screamed: 4 points

Does your car go to the mechanic's shop for routine maintenance more often than you go to your health center for routine health prevention?

Yes: 2 points

Do you spend more time in your car each week than with your . . .

Spouse or best friend? Yes: 1 point
Kids? Yes: 1 point

Do you spend more money on your car each year than on your spouse or parents?

Yes: 1 point

Do you drive less than one mile . . .

Once per week: 1 point
2–4 times per week: 2 points
5 times or more per week: 3 points

Have you *ever* driven to your mailbox?

Yes: 1 point

CAR SCORE

0–3 points: You are in command of your car (or perhaps you don't have one).
3–6 points: You are car-centric.
7–10 points: You are car-dependent.
11 points+: You're glued to your car seat.

It does not take much time to reverse excessive car use. Move from your car seat to your feet for an extra 18 minutes every day, and you will change the world!

8

THE CHAIRMAN'S VISION

CAN *HOMO SEDENTARIUS* GO FROM BIRTH TO DEATH WITH-
out getting to his or her feet? Unless we reverse lethal sitting, the
next scenario depicts what we'll become.

THE CHAIRMAN'S FANTASY

If The Chairman has his way, *Homo sedentarius* will go from crib
to coffin without taking a step. Let's look into his vision of the
future.

After birth, Baby Chari rests in her crib. Soon she learns to
sit in baby's first chair (Life Stage I chair). She is not discouraged
from learning to walk, but since there isn't any purpose in doing
so, Chari's baby chair is designed for optimum comfort. In order
to encourage (and teach) the child to sit still, from the age of
two Chari is handed a lightweight tablet with an infinite supply
of moving pictures, sounds and screen-based stimuli; Chari is
happy to endlessly sit still and stare.

Chari's parents divorce when she is age three, and Dad becomes just a press-here away on the tablet. When Chari's dad is
not actually available to interact with his child, a programmable

bot with his face tells Chari (via the interface) that he loves his daughter. Chari, immersed in educational software, learns to read and speak in her Life Stage II chair. Because all parents in each country use the same learning software, there is a similarity in how all children learn to speak—and so the death of individuality begins. Individuality is a curse because the educational software systems cater to the average.

Sadly Chari's grandparents die (they are Gen 1 victims of sitting disease). Because data show the developmental benefit of grandparents and family, Chari is assigned two virtual grandparents with appropriate skin tone, language and religious programming. The computer interface has advanced so that Chari can smell virtual Grandma Jenny's perfume and feel the touch of virtual Grandpa Jack through robotically controlled hands attached to Chari's Life Stage II chair.

By the age of five, Chari is accustomed to interact with her parents online even when they are in the same home. Because Chari's mother and (divorced) father are often busy, virtual Grandma Jenny often sings and strokes Chari to sleep. Virtual Grandpa Jack tells Chari a story every day at exactly 4 p.m.; the story aligns with Chari's programmed culture. It never crosses Chari's mind that she can't remember physically meeting her grandparents; after all, she has never actually met her 117 friends or 29 cousins.

Soon little Chari is ready to go to school—virtually, from her Life Stage III chair. The virtual schooling system is superior to antiquated concrete systems because lessons are standardized, school buildings are unnecessary and all children have a nice, culturally sifted cohort of friends. Using a mix-modulator algorithm, Chari's mixture of real and computer-simulated friends guarantees a perfect race, income-status and sex-based mix in her class. The chair-based educational experience is enhanced with surround-sound class noise, self-pacing and a grading system controlled by a computer that adjusts how grades are given based on levels of Self-Esteem Opiate (SEO) in Chari's blood.

During the 12 years of Chari's chair-based education, socialization is encouraged and advanced using behavioral algorithms; studies show that this system is superior to skin-based friendship because (a) there are no transmissible diseases; (b) there are no hurtful interactions, such as bullying or negative stereotyping, that lower SEO levels; (c) Chari never uses marijuana—unlike one in three high school students in the old school system—and (d) she is immune from risk of teen pregnancy—unlike one in ten girls in the old skin-based system.[1]

Although perhaps difficult to imagine, child socialization now occurs exclusively through electronic screen-based interactions. Children list their friends on computer systems; they may not have met many of those friends, and some do not actually exist. Chari learns and socializes entirely from her chair; her environment is sterile but safe.

What about sitting death: the health consequences of sitting too much? What does the future hold for young Chari in this regard? The international concern regarding the epidemic of childhood diabetes and escalating rates of childhood hypertension will no longer be a worry. This is because, from the age of two, Chari is given a polypill that adjusts the body's response to hormones such as insulin and also works on the brain to slow down signals that might encourage excessive levels of daily activity. DNA analysis enables the polypill to be individualized for different children's needs. For example, a child prone to moodiness receives a polypill with a little amphetamine. Chari's pill contains an SEO booster, so she is immune to any self-doubt. An excessively imaginative child, in contrast, may receive a polypill with a hint of benzodiazepine to make her easier to teach. Importantly, all children get a polypill that protects them from excessive disease burden and emotional responsiveness. Medication for life. If you think this concept too futuristic, to date more than 200 scientific articles have been written about polypills.[2]

At the end of Chari's chair-based education, she will virtually attend graduation with real and bot friends; online Chari will receive her congratulatory handshake from the principal using the robotic arm attached to her Life Stage III chair and a hug from her absent father using the same technology.

Young-adult Chari enters college much in the same way as school—from her chair. As of 2012, CorpWatch, a nonprofit research group (www.corpwatch.org), estimated the online college industry to be worth $650 billion in the United States alone—about the gross domestic product of Thailand.[3] By the time Chari is in college, virtual universities are viewed as superior because they access leading teachers from around the world; land-based universities carry the overhead of concrete and cannot compete. By the time Chari graduates college, she has upgraded to her Life Stage IV chair.

Graduate Chari enters the workplace and moves to her own apartment. Chari is a ChUPY (chair-based urban professional youth); she not only works from the desk in her apartment but orders food and arranges apartment cleaning from her desk as well. Groceries arrive from a virtual supermarket. Movie theaters deliver content through net streaming, including scent streaming and pheromone blasts so that viewers can directly experience the emotions depicted. Movies and television are careful not to depict active people in order not to appear unrealistic. Movie stars are rarely seen to rise from their chairs; sitting is in vogue.

The advantage of acquiring a life partner without leaving one's apartment is that your computer-based photograph can be manipulated to show you in the best light. Armed with an array of beautification photographs and downloaded scripts, Chari mingles on virtual dating platforms. She is erudite and intelligent, and her chair-based virtual chat is aided by intelligence bots. When Chari is spotted by another eligible ChUPY, drinks can be virtually purchased for her and delivered to her apartment; that way she never needs to drink and drive. Using the robotic arms attached to her Life Stage IV chair, controlled touching can occur and unwanted advances, rejected. With the correct scent dissemination hardware, Chari's perfume can be transmitted across the virtual bar and the potential partner turned on (or off) as Chari deems right. And so the classic bar pickup can be achieved from one chair to another. Gone are excessively pushy men and coy women; also gone are nights drinking alone because robotic dates can fill in should people not be available.

The first dinner date is similarly orchestrated. Chari need only pick the menu and the food will be hand delivered to her date's apartment. Her date may chivalrously remotely select wine, which Chari will similarly receive in her chair. Awkward dinner conversation is easily prevented using date-specific bot-generated content. Importantly, if things don't work out, all Chari needs to do is hit the off button.

The notion of virtual sex may seem inhuman to any person who has indulged in the skin-based system. Nonetheless, virtual sex is already a $70-billion-a-year business. Virtual toys, sex chat and video are universal. Chari will be able to indulge in sexual activities with her partner via voice and visual connection, transmitted robotic arm commands, Internet scent transmission and plug-in stimulators. If Chari's date happens to be a male, his arousal is easily secured using the robotic hand attached to his computer. If Chari's date is female, different attachments for the date's robotic arm can be used. Without leaving their chairs, the young couple can "get serious" and wed—virtually; everyone will be able to attend the wedding. Chari will be able to work, eat, sleep and marry without ever leaving her favorite Life Stage IV chair.

In 2013, London's *Daily Mail* reported, "One in ten modern couples live separately because they feel 'emotionally safer' if they keep their independence."[4] Chari and her husband (or wife) live separately too. When it comes time for our emotionally safe young couple to procreate, Chari still does not need to leave her chair. Using the robotic arm (and some postmarital plug-ins), her husband can provide a sample of his DNA that is FedExed to Chari. If Chari's spouse is a woman, the couple can browse sperm options from Internet providers. Chari, without leaving the chair in her apartment, will then inject the mailed sperm inside of her. The Life Stage IV chair has a base that is removed for impregnation and birthing. An alternate is simply to order children though Always_shopping.com. (Better children come if you have Always_shopping Prime.) And so the cycle of chair-life begins again.

Just as adults can spend their entire work lives in their chairs, raise their children and never leave their apartment, retirement is similarly chair-based. When it's all done, the Life Stage V chair flattens out to become a coffin.

All the technologies I have described in my chair-based nightmare exist. In New York, Los Angeles, San Francisco and other major cities, it is already possible to live entirely from your apartment chair. Although my nightmare may seem ludicrous, what I describe is horribly close to what we have right now: a sedentary, stifled populace, isolated from each other, living in chairs in front of computer screens and slowly dying from lethal sitting.

If we are going to change direction, how do we begin?

PART III

OUST THE CHAIRMAN

The Solution Revolution

9

SOLUTIONS

Why Do We Need Them?

THE AVERAGE AMERICAN SITS 13 HOURS PER DAY; 86 PER-
cent of Americans sit all day at work and 68 percent hate it.[1] The
health and psychological harm of excess sitting is indisputable.
So why the status quo? Why are Americans and the majority of
people in the developed world stuck on their bottoms? Why is
Western society chair addicted?

There is an extraordinary paradox about lethal sitting. If sitting is so bad for our bodies, brains and souls, surely the solution
is simple: get up. But whenever I talk to my patients about the
idea of decreasing their sit time by 2 hours and 15 minutes each
day, they are overwhelmed by the challenge. However, we know
from the science that (a) people can, without changing their environment or job description, get up and move for 2 hours and
15 minutes more than before and (b) the natural human capacity
to move is twice as much as even active Americans move.[2] We
can do it.

If sedentariness is so dangerous and reversing it is so easy,
surely we should have solved the problem by now. That is the

paradox; what seems so straightforward—getting up—is in reality hard. Escaping the chair sentence requires the invention and validation of effective chair-escape solutions.

The NEAT lab has tested hundreds of solutions to reverse lethal sitting. But for any human being, there is a moment of truth—where each person has to decide between two courses of action. One way keeps you in your chair. The other way is to take the *necessary* risk and get up.

The ground beneath the four legs of our chairs feels firm—solid, secure. But it is not. Society is fundamentally ill at ease. Go into any office with its hundreds of chair-containing cubicles and you can sense the malaise. The ground beneath our chairs is rumbling. Before we can resolve sedentariness and escape the chair sentence, we must look deep beneath the foundations—not society's but our own.

THE STORIES WE TELL OURSELVES ARE NOT NECESSARILY TRUE

Throughout our lives, we invent a voice in our heads that talks to us all day long. The stories I tell myself are often untruthful. Just recently I told myself I could *never* learn to bake bread; I was wrong. It was dead simple.

Often clients battling obesity tell themselves that they are unattractive and unworthy; the data suggest they tell themselves this many times each hour.[3] This continuous internal narrative can be positive as well; however, most people criticize rather than praise themselves.

Culture dramatically impacts the voices in our heads. Much of our internal storytelling is based on stories pulled from generations before us. In Japan, for example, people's internal voices have a far more Japanese cultural feel than do those of Japanese people living in the United States.[4] When I was working with children who had been forced into prostitution in Mumbai, they told me about how they create stories about alternate lives that fill their heads. These inner voices separate them from the horror of their reality. We each have an internal voice; it is a part of being human. So, like our clothing and cooking, these internal voices are impacted by the environment in which we exist.

INSIDE THE AMERICAN HEAD

An important part of the American inner voice is a story we create regarding what happiness is—what we should aspire to. In the internal American voice—the voice inside our collective head—"wealth" and "happiness" are synonymous. Implicit in that narrative is that winning (wealth and success) means beating out the competition. Winning is drilled into us in preschool.

I remember the intensity of the many years my daughter spent in competitive gymnastics from the age of ten on. Training was compulsory three times a week, meets were held around the country and the only goal was to win. In the broader US society, winning is the goal. Winning is success. Success is money. Money is happiness. The American economy is based on a money-is-happiness mentality: Shop till you drop, no end to spend, the winner gets stuff.

A professor who teaches consumerism and marketing explained to me that the art of marketing is to connect the buying of an object to mortality. Car advertisements, for example, often show high-speed drives or family groups—in different ways, both allude to our mortality.

Inside the collective American head, owning objects correlates to living, so owning more possessions correlates with prolonged life—consumerism becomes the elixir of living. The most successful people are the richest, and so potentially live the longest. This idea extends beyond theory—rich people generally *do* live longer because they have better healthcare and health-promoting facilities. However, a part of winning is that somebody else has to lose. In order to be the best, you have to beat out someone else. Inevitably winning is isolating—it is all about getting to the top. The trouble is, the top is a lonely place.

TRIBAL LIVING

There is a Native American story about a tribe. The tribe functioned well; hunters hunted, gatherers harvested, explorers explored and homemakers managed homes; the elderly, sick and children were cared for. There was enough for everyone. One day the number one hunter thought to himself, "I am the best hunter. I kill the most. Why should I share my bounty with everyone else?" And so number one hunter built himself a hut on top of a mountain and kept everything he caught for himself.

Soon other hunters followed suit, and one after another went to live alone at the top of mountains. The tribe could not carry on; the elderly and the sick soon perished, and the homemakers and children had to flee.

But here is what happened to the hunters living on the mountaintops. Number one hunter gorged himself and gained so much fat he could no longer hunt. He died of sickness—the medicine man had left long ago. Other hunters, without craftspeople to make their spears and arrows or the value of shared knowledge, were not as skilled as they thought and soon failed. They died hungry.

The tribe exists as much for the strong as for the weak. The need for excess serves no one. In native cultures, people who live in spaces larger than they require are viewed as having a spiritual disorder akin to madness.

Plato described the essence of society as being the need to acquire a critical mass of people and then to develop a cohesiveness based on reciprocity of skills (e.g., a doctor) and allocation of tasks (e.g., security duty) among different people. Interestingly, this societal cohesiveness occurs in the animal world.

I used to live in rural Minnesota. As winter froze in, I would watch the flocks of birds fly out. It intrigued me as how they seem to all know which way to swerve and turn, hundreds of birds together. What actually happens is that within a single wing beat, birds adjust their flights to follow the flock. If you watch a flock, you will never see one bird fly away by itself; they're always together. They never go so fast that one will be left behind, and they never go so slow that they freeze in the Minnesota winter. Think of families of penguins, schools of fish, beehives and ant mounds, and communities of chimpanzees. Cohesiveness is in living beings' DNA. If the DNA of all these species is encoded to purposely retain connectivity as a group, so too must the DNA of humans. Humans are built to cluster together.

Millions of humans sit in chairs all day long in order to be as monetarily productive as possible. Advertisements that prod our sense of mortality collectively seduce us to buy unnecessary objects. The bitter irony is that we have put our mortality on the line by sitting for long enough to buy these objects. These chairs we sit on, alone and lonely, for 13 hours a day are killing us!

10

INVENT!

Underwear Solutions

TECHNOLOGY IS A PART OF THE CAUSE OF LETHAL SITTING, but it is an inevitable part of the solution as well. How can technology help reverse lethal sitting?

As I mentioned in chapter 2, we used magic underwear to track sitting and NEAT (nonexercise activity thermogenesis) activity in our research studies. Each set of underwear cost $7,000; disseminating the underwear nationwide would be cost prohibitive. To expand our work, we needed a physical activity measuring device that was inexpensive and could be used by potentially thousands of people. I began to look in the scientific literature.

In 1999, long before cell phones were commonplace, I found a device called the Tracmor. The Tracmor was a technology that allowed daily movement to be accurately measured minute-by-minute for days on end.[1] A decade later, a host of devices would come onto the market to do the same thing (the Fitbit®, Gruve®, Nike+ FuelBand® and Kam® devices are examples), but the Tracmor was not only far ahead of its time, it also had been scientifically validated.

The only scientific group that used the Tracmor was in the Netherlands. I wrote to one of the lead professors, whom I'll call Professor Fartoobusy. I sent a batch of emails—no response. I tried to telephone—he seemed to be perpetually unavailable. Becoming progressively more frustrated, I sent a FedEx letter. No response. After a total of nine FedExes, it was time for action, time *to get up*.

Without an appointment but in a torrent of passion, I headed off to a small town in the Netherlands where Professor Fartoobusy worked. It was amusing to enter his office unannounced. I walked in pulling my suitcase behind me. His secretary looked me up and down and asked in perfect, clipped English who I was. I explained that I was Dr. Levine from Mayo Clinic. She said, "You have to have an appointment—the professor doesn't just see anyone." I answered, "Please just tell the professor that I have flown from the United States to visit him." She called through my request; then a heated exchange in Dutch occurred. Fartoobusy, long legged and gaunt, bounded out of his office. His cheeks were red, and he was flustered as he said, "Dr. Levine, I was just about to reply to your letters. What are you doing here?"

I explained that I urgently needed to get a device that would help crush the chair sentence. Fartoobusy smiled and offered me coffee. We walked together, and he explained that he was not in charge of this technology; Professor Klaus Westerterp was. He was in Maastricht, several hours' drive away. I thanked Fartoobusy and asked him to call Professor Westerterp and tell him that I was on my way.

It was a long but fast drive to Maastricht. Physically, Professor Klaus Westerterp was almost the opposite of Fartoobusy. He was five foot six and had shoulder-length, sandy brown hair, a gentle smile and was dressed in jeans and an open-necked shirt. He had heard of my coming—the impassioned scientist who had flown from America unannounced to meet Fartoobusy. I liked Klaus immediately. He grasped my hand. "What an unexpected pleasure," he said. It was the beginning of a decade-long friendship. I left Maastricht with five of his Tracmor units.

The Tracmor units looked as if they had been built in a laboratory. They were clumsily put together, each consisting of a large gray box about the size of a soda can connected via a wire to a small, 2-inch brown resin square. The gray box contained the electronics that stored the data, but the innovation was inside the brown resin square. Hidden inside the resin square were three acceleration sensors (accelerometers) pointing in different directions. Each of the three accelerometers captured movement in one direction (forward/backward, left/right or up/down). When the resin square was taped to a person's back, the Tracmor could detect if a person was walking or motionless. The Tracmor unit allowed us for the first time to measure how free-living people went about their daily lives, whether burning calories while moving (NEAT) or being sedentary.

The scientific community had proven that chair addiction caused obesity and a host of medical problems; the Tracmor was a technology that measured motion and sedentariness while people went about their normal daily lives far away from the laboratory. This breakthrough was critical because it enabled me to better understand how sedentary people behave in the real world and to assess what interventions are best to reverse lethal sitting. The Tracmor was excellent for scientific studies in free-living people but it was not ready for the mass market. I needed a technological approach that could reach millions.

At that time, 15 years ago, the music industry was being reinvented. Every other word was "iPod." I recognized that the best way to make moving cool was to integrate our ideas into the iPod. I wrote to Tony Fadell, the president at Apple in charge of the iPod division. In a brief telephone conversation, I explained to him that I wanted to adapt the magic underwear technology for the iPod. I expected him to laugh and hang up. He laughed but he didn't hang up; the NEAT lab was invited to Apple. I realized that we were not being invited to Apple to make a scientific presentation. This was business. This was our chance to get the chair sentence message out, to begin a mass campaign against The Chairman.

Since the NEAT lab was going to visit one of the greatest self-marketing companies in the world, I decided that we needed to meet power with power. I needed to hire a media consultant. I needed Adam Taub. Like the Monty Python actors and Sacha Baron Cohen, Adam wrote for the Cambridge University comedy troupe called Footlights.[2] Adam had started off at Cambridge as a science major and then switched to law. After graduation, he became a production manager at Intel and then a prominent patent attorney. Finally, he opened his own marketing company. Within a year, he was scripting for television and running international corporate media events. Adam could help me script my pitch to Apple.

A week later, Adam had flown from London to the NEAT lab at Mayo. He needed to understand the science. He bought a bottle of wine and took me out at midnight on a remote lake in a canoe. When the bottle was empty, he asked me what I wanted from him. I told him I needed to wake up America and then the world. The chair is killing us. In the middle of the lake with the sun rising, I stood up in the canoe and shouted, "I need a revolution."

Adam wrote scripts for the Apple presentation. We rehearsed as if we were actors; he corrected gestures, body postures and delivery. After a week we were ready, and three of us flew to Cupertino for the Apple presentation: Adam Taub, Paul (the master engineer) and me.

At Apple, we were ushered into a small conference room, and several of their technical and businesspeople entered. We prepared our stage. I sweated profusely in my suit—as if I were about to go live on Broadway! Tony Fadell entered last. This man was head of the whole iPod program. He had a giant smile and emanated "cool" like cologne. "Doctor, it's such a pleasure to have you at Apple," he said. He was a man you instantly liked. "So what have you got to show us?"

Adam was master of ceremonies; he gave the introduction. Next came Paul, who explained the technology, its capabilities and why we needed millions of people to engage in monitoring their daily NEAT levels. Then it was my turn. I began to explain the magic underwear technology and started a striptease, removing my suit jacket, tie, shirt, shoes, socks and suit pants. I was wearing the technology under my business clothes. At this point, Tony stopped smiling and looked as if he had entered a new reality. By this time I had stripped down to the magic underwear complete with wires and flashing lights, wearing only swimming trunks beneath it. The room was utterly silent. Everyone looked at Tony, who said, "You really are Dr. Levine from the Mayo Clinic, right?" I nodded.

Tony walked over to me, shook my hand and said, "If this is what all of our meetings are going to be like, we've *got* to work together. I have never quite seen a presentation like this before!"

A year later, the first mass movement sensing system was launched collaboratively between Apple and Nike (Nikeplus: http://www.apple.com/ipod/nike/). Shoe sensors synced with iPods, and soon millions of people had begun to measure their daily activity levels. For the first time, people could self-monitor their daily activity.

The NEAT lab had changed. We no longer worked in a laboratory focused on Ivory Tower research. We had morphed into something different. We had a mission: to free the chair-sentenced masses from their sedentary servitude. The measurement revolution had begun.

MEMS: MICRO MACHINES SMALLER THAN A PERIOD

MEMS (micro electro-mechanical systems) technology consists of microchips the size of pencil erasers. MEMS accelerometer microchips cost only cents and can directly measure human movement.[3] Inside the chips are microscopic teeth that slide back and forth depending on the amount of movement a person makes; the amount of movement is converted into an electrical signal. MEMS accelerometer chips have been incorporated into devices such as the Fitbit®, Gruve® device, LUMOback®, Nike+ FuelBand® and Adidas miCoach® system. They've enabled millions of people to measure their sedentariness and track their chair escape.

I'm often asked which of the various activity-tracking devices is best. MEMS chips are valid and reliable. What is more important is how well the device attaches to the body. Research studies demonstrate that the most reliable data are obtained when MEMS accelerometers are placed against the skin on a part of the body connected to the trunk, such as the base of the spine.[4] Although wrist and shoe devices can deliver crude data, they cannot detect when your bottom is on the chair.

Regardless of whether you buy an activity tracker for yourself or your dog, most Americans are carrying a MEMS accelerometer chip without realizing. There is a MEMS chip inside your smartphone. Here, the MEMS accelerometer is used to change the screen from portrait to landscape when you turn the phone.

When the first iPhone came out in 2007, I brought one to the laboratory and hacked into the signal from its MEMS chip. The accuracy was comparable to our research-grade magic underwear. At the time, apps were new. I needed an activity app. To create one, I telephoned Professor Ioannis Pavlidis.

Ioannis comes from Greece. Not only does he run the Computational Physiology Lab at the University of Houston, but he also spontaneously recites philosophy and poetry. My call found him in a coffee shop. I explained that I needed an app that detected the chair sentence. He listened, quoted a South American poet and hung up.

In six weeks, Ioannis had written the first app that enabled people to track their daily NEAT activity using their iPhone without buying any special equipment. He called it Walk n' Play.

He validated the app in our lab and released it at a national conference.[5] The press picked it up, and *Business Week* selected it as one of its favorite apps. Two days later the University of Houston servers were under siege. Twenty-eight thousand users were measuring their sedentariness ten times each second.

If, during my PhD work, I had said to my mentor, Marsha Morgan, that one day I could measure human calorie burn in 28,000 people every tenth of a second for weeks at a time, she would have said I was delusional. But it happened; the app with 28,000 users had cost us nothing. Technologies driven by MEMS accelerometer chips enable potentially millions of people to self-monitor their daily activity.[6]

Today there are numerous apps for measuring physical activity, sitting and sedentariness. These types of MEMS-monitoring tools render it feasible to assess and ultimately prompt the reversal of chair addiction.

YOU AIN'T SEEN NOTHING YET

More technologies are coming that have the potential to profoundly impact sitting disease.[7] Wearable technologies are coming to the fore. For example, several designs for bras containing multiple health sensors exist. New types of band-aids will inform wearers via a transmitted text message when they have been sitting for too long and need to get up. Other skin-worn sensors can sense your level of dehydration, stress and sleep so that you are best informed on how to win your tech-savvy quest for active health.

But don't think that these technologies are just for you; your pooch can have his or her sitting measured as well, and you will be informed via a downloadable app if you are ignoring your dog's walking needs. There is even a system where you can see how active your pet fish has been!

Tremendous technology developments are afoot in the medical space. I foresee that every home will have a medical hub that will sync medical data, such as blood pressure, weight, blood sugar, electrocardiogram and sweat concentrations, to your remote medical center so that instead of your health being assessed a few times a year, it will be sensed and acted on almost continuously.

The cell phone will become a portable health hub; daily life will become more game-ified so that actively moving around your city becomes more fun. Also, I anticipate that social media will integrate body sensors so that you can "Like" the activity level of a friend and nudge another friend who is sitting too much. "Health nets" will connect millions of people who want to escape their chair sentences—together.

FRIENDLY TECHNOLOGY?

Labor-saving technologies of various types impact us every hour we are awake. From the moment we wake up, we look at the electronic clock that, 50 years ago, would have been wound by hand. We move from our beds, press the TV remote control to switch on the morning news, access our tablets to check our mail (rather than walk to the mailbox), grind coffee in a machine and then brew it in another machine. We can switch on our lights without touching them. Our homes are heated by touching a switch rather than cutting wood or shoveling coal. Water comes from a tap—not hand pulled by a well. From our heated homes we might jump in our cars, grab breakfast at a drive-through and take an elevator up to our offices. Just a generation ago, people did every single one of these activities by hand or on foot. Today, on a given morning, we can utilize more than 70 labor-saving devices without breaking a sweat!

I was recently taunted in a National Institutes of Health conference as being the godfather of the anti-chair mafia. You might think that the godfather of the anti-chair mafia would seek the extermination of all labor-saving devices; you would be wrong. I do not advocate reversing progress. Labor-saving devices are here to stay. But we need to think about these tools of convenience differently. What these tools actually do is free up our minds, arms and legs to do useful things, like go for a walk with a friend, take an art class, volunteer, play piano or learn tai chi. Ultimately it comes down to how we use these technologies, for evil or good.

11

WORK!

Office Solutions

NEW ADVANCES FROM OLD LESSONS

In the 1960s almost half of jobs in the United States required a moderate amount of physical activity (for example, running a printing press or working on a production line). Since then that number has fallen drastically. Now, 80 percent of US workers sit on their bottoms throughout their workday, and over the next ten years the number of chair-sentenced workers is expected to increase even more.[1] What is more concerning is that 68 percent of workers hate sitting all day.[2]

This is not just a US phenomenon; similar progressive declines in occupational nonexercise activity thermogenesis (NEAT) are occurring in the United Kingdom, Brazil, China and India,[3] and in these countries, the situation is projected to worsen as well. Currently, more than half of the population of the developed and developing world work seated in front of computer screens.[4]

The health impact of the workplace chair sentence will send a shiver up your spine. In 1958 there were less than 2 million people in the United States with diabetes. That number has increased 17-fold; today in America 26 million Americans have diabetes and 80 million Americans have prediabetes (high blood sugars), forewarning of a tsunami of diabetes.[5] One in three American adults already has high blood pressure,[6] greatly increasing the risk for heart disease and stroke.

Diabetes and high blood pressure alone cost the US health-care system $268 billion. That money is paid predominantly by working Americans and their insurers. Add to this the costs of back pain, depression, cancer, cardiovascular disease and poor productivity and you realize that lethal sitting is impactful on the economic viability of the United States.[7] The CDC estimates that these types of conditions explain 75 percent of US healthcare costs.[8] If ever there has been a time to think differently about how we work, now is that time.

I am not claiming that the chair sentence explains the entire catalog of workplace woe, but it explains a lot of it. If we can find sustainable ways to get people up while at work, there are millions of lives and hundreds of billions of dollars that can be saved. Is it possible to work productively and effectively but *not* sit all day? *Yes.*

CHANGING PLACES

In the 1980s, workplace scientists from Japan best demonstrated the power of workplace design to impact productivity.[9] They considered two factories; one had globe light bulbs and the other, strip fluorescent lights. All the scientists did was switch the lighting around between the two factories. The altered sensory stimulation was sufficient to affect behavior, and productivity improved in both factories. In 2010 researchers at the Carlson School of Management hung posters on office walls that depicted people being active. They found that office workers moved more as a result.[10]

Lynn Bui, a young worker in Umea, Sweden, had read about lethal sitting. In her office, the desks had adjustable heights and could be used sitting or standing. She had observed that, almost without exception, the 137 desks were generally in the lowered position and workers sat. Lynn undertook an audacious two-week experiment: She removed all 137 chairs and put them in the basement. She put up posters to explain the dangers of sitting and why she had removed the chairs. For the next two weeks, Lynn carefully monitored the responses.

A few people were angry and immediately retrieved their chairs from the basement; others were confused but decided to try standing for a few hours; others took chairs from nearby meeting rooms and substituted them for their desk chairs; some moved to rooms with chairs.

Many workers, however, decided to give the experiment a go, some for the entire two weeks. Of the 137 removed chairs, 44 chairs were returned to the office floor after the first day, 70 after the second day, 99 after the first week and 103 after two weeks. After two weeks, 34 chairs remained in the basement.

"The experiment worked better than expected," Lynn explained. "Previously normative behavior had changed. It no longer looked weird to stand, knowing that others were also doing it. Clusters began to form in different areas . . . Some groups mostly sat, others alternated, and others stood as much as they could. Some people took the challenge for two weeks. 'It's not so hard after a while,' one reported." The experiment, Bui concluded, "provided the scale of interruption necessary for people to generate a memorable reflection on sitting."

THE ANTI-CHAIR: BIRTH OF THE TREADMILL DESK

The idea of treadmill desks is simple: (1) Get a treadmill and place a stand over it at about chest height; (2) put your computer and mouse on the stand; (3) switch on the treadmill at 1 mph; and (4) voilà! Walk and work. Treadmill desks have spread around the world; manufacturers told me that as of 2011, at least 50,000 of them were in use.

The inspiration behind the treadmill desk occurred in 2000, when the two parts of my life collided—professional and personal. In the lab, data were streaming in from our studies. Lean people do not sit. The personal part was harder to swallow.

I came to the United States from Britain at age 24 and soon adopted the American male archetype: Homer Simpson. Getting home from work at six, exhausted, the remainder of my evening would be spent on the sofa watching TV: *The Simpsons*, *Seinfeld* and sports. I played with my small daughters but only while on the sofa with a bag of chips between my legs. One day my wife said, "Jim, you've put on weight. You need to get up and work out." I'd gained 30 pounds. I hated the gym.

The following day, I sat in my office and thought, "How can I get an extra 2 hours and 15 minutes of walking into my day?" I realized that it had to be during the workday. I concluded, "Treadmill plus desk equals walk and work." We had a gifted psychologist, Leslie Olson, working in the lab who also happened to be a farmer, musician and carpenter. I explained my idea to Leslie, and we headed to the hospital basement, where broken furniture was deposited for parts. There we found an old patient table—one of those adjustable ones that slides under a patient's bed and can be raised and lowered. It was easily repaired with an Allen wrench and duct tape. Next we needed a treadmill, so I looked online; a barely used Sears model was on sale for $350. On the way home, I picked it up and put it in my truck.

After my children and wife were asleep, I snuck back to work. I dragged the treadmill up to my office and, using a reciprocating saw, cut off the steel sides. I slid the duct-taped patient tray table under the treadmill base and moved my computer onto it. And so by 2 a.m. the first treadmill desk was operational. I stepped on board and within a few minutes I had answered my first email while striding along at 3 mph. Soon I was tired and realized that you can't walk and work at 3 mph, so I went back to the data. If I wanted to emulate the activity level of a lean person, I needed to understand the speed at which lean people walk.

Using Big Data number-crunching analytics, I pulled our data on 10,000 walking episodes in lean people. The average speed of all walks was only 1.1 mph. As dawn rose, I was walking along at 1.1 mph and working. The treadmill desk was born.

At first people thought I was crazy—literally. Complaints came from people in my work unit that this was a disruptive idea, but on I walked. I saw changes in myself immediately; I stopped surfing the Internet in the afternoon, I went home with more energy and started to play with my kids—off the sofa at last!

A few years after this, I had a call from the *New York Times*. The health editor, Denise Grady, wanted to talk. Grady's calm, well-researched insightfulness struck me immediately, and I invited her to visit the lab. "I was hoping you'd say that," she replied. Grady visited for two days. She probed our equipment, the data and the concepts. "It's not exercise," she said. "We call it nonexercise activity thermogenesis—NEAT," I replied. "The calories we burn in everyday living."

I explained how people with obesity sit 2 hours and 15 minutes a day more than lean people living in the same environments. Grady asked, "So what's the answer?" I explained that we have to find ways to give people who are battling the bulge (i.e., me!) a fighting chance. I told her that we have to integrate walking—an extra 2 hours and 15 minutes of walking a day—throughout the day if we are to win. The treadmill desk allowed just that. You could stay at work—never leave work—and walk an extra 2 hours and 15 minutes a day, no sweat. When Grady published a two-page spread in the *New York Times* about NEAT, the concept erupted.[11]

I spoke with media outlets around the world. I have long disagreed with many of my colleagues who deride the press for inaccuracy. If you are trying to get a new idea out, you have to explain it to the media. It takes hours, and there's a lot of repetition, but it's worth it. The awareness of the sitting disease spread worldwide.

Home-based workers took to the treadmill desk concept with passion. They sent me photographs of treadmill desks made from cardboard boxes, reconfigured shelving units and homemade wood-framed structures. Most people worked on treadmills, but some used exercise bicycles or gliding machines that mimic cross-country skiing. Reports started to come in; some users lost 45, 50 or 70 pounds, and others experienced decreased back pain or improved sleep. All the treadmill desk users I heard from felt better and more productive, walking while working. Eventually treadmill desk users coalesced in social networking sites, and bloggers blogged from their newfound treadmill desk bliss.

These self-rigged treadmill desks were great for people working from home. But this approach would not work in corporate offices where corporations assume liability for workplace injuries. If the treadmill desk was going to break into the corporate world, I had to convert my duct-taped patient table and sawn-up treadmill into a professional unit.

FROM DUCT TAPE TO PRODUCT

The advance of the treadmill desk to an international furniture sensation came though my relationship with Steelcase. Leaders at Steelcase had read the *New York Times* article and wanted to know more; they asked for me to visit them. In a way, I was about to meet the enemy—one of the leading manufacturers of chairs. One of Sun Tzu's 13 principles of war, written 2,500 years ago, is this: "The most efficient style of warfare is to destroy the coalitions against you and forge alliances on your behalf." Off I went to Steelcase.

Details, the subdivision of Steelcase I worked with, was led by Bud Klipa. White-haired, broad and tall, Bud is the essence of leadership—a man who inspires others. He was charming yet persuasive. His small team built the first commercial treadmill desks in 2007. The Steelcase desk fit the standard office cubicle footprint, and the treadmill was geared for slow speed (1–1.5

mph is the ideal walk-and-work speed) and went to a maximum speed of 2 mph; that way no one could fly off and hurt himself or herself. Most important, the treadmill desk was beautiful; the lines were clean, and the entire structure was rigid. It was time to test the idea in the mainstream.

Steelcase launched the desk in its New York showroom on Broadway. A few hours after the unveiling, Diane Sawyer invited us to demo the desks on *Good Morning America*.[12] At 6 a.m. the following day, I helped the Steelcase team assemble four desks in the television studio and then stood by.

An hour later Diane Sawyer and Deborah Roberts got up from their chairs. It was time to film the treadmill desk segment. It would go out live. I gasped. Both women were wearing high heels. The world started to spin. I always suggest that women wear tennis shoes when using a treadmill desk; never heels. When I suggested this to Ms. Sawyer, she looked at me, smiled kindly and stepped on to a desk. "How does this work?" she asked. Two other presenters stepped forward. Soon four national anchors *in heels* were walking on my desks. I knew that if one of them even stumbled, the NEAT revolution was over and the desk concept would be caput.

My career flashed before my eyes. The cameras went live and 32 inches of heels clipped through the piece without falter. Deborah Roberts concluded, "This is a lifesaver," and the treadmill desk was launched.

THE MYSTERY OF THE EMPTY GYM

I was once asked to consult for a major US corporation. It had a four-story, square-shaped office building. At the two corners of every floor, the company had installed, at great expense, small gyms. I was asked to visit the corporation to determine why no one used these mini-gyms.

I was offered a multiday consultancy to understand what was going on; it took me less than an hour to discover the answer.

On the third floor, I walked into an office adjacent to one of these mini-gyms. A handful of young employees worked intently, heads down, at their desks.

I coughed loudly; three looked up. I asked, "Why do you guys never use these cool mini-gyms?" One snorted and went straight back to work. A young Asian woman said, "If we go there, it looks like we're not working."

"How about your lunchtimes?" I asked.

She raised her eyebrows. "What lunchtimes?"

No one used these gyms because there was a uniform belief (the collective consciousness) that if you exercised in the workplace, (a) you were not at your desk and (b) you were not serious about your work.

You can have all the treadmill desks in the world, activity monitors up the wazoo, interns who hide your chairs and on and on, *but* unless the corporate culture permits and encourages chairlessness, you are sentenced to lethal sitting.

In stark contrast to this, when I met the chief executive of Nike, our meeting was held in the corporate gym on two treadmills.

Culture is critical.

CULTURE IN THE IVORY COAST (VIA ROME)

In 2001 I wanted to understand how culture affected sitting. Having decided that the best way to get at this would be to study disparate cultures across the world, I contacted the Food and Agricultural Organization (FAO) at the United Nations. I sent just one email to the general inquiries website. I explained who I was and that I wanted to understand the role of culture on sedentariness. The next day Dr. Barbara Burlingame replied, explaining that FAO in Rome had been conducting in-depth studies in the Ivory Coast, but the work had prematurely halted. One of the most senior scientists at FAO, Barbara needed someone to pick up the project; a week later I was in Rome.

FAO is at the top of Circus Maximus, where charioteers used to race in ancient Rome. I stayed opposite the Vatican and walked through the city to FAO. When I arrived, security called Dr. Burlingame. I waited and soon Barbara whirled into my life, trailing a long blue-and-red chiffon cape. We drank coffee on the roof overlooking the Coliseum and Rome's Seven Hills. With that view, it was difficult to concentrate on work. Barbara explained that enormous amounts of data had been gathered from the Ivory Coast, but with the death of one of the lead investigators, it was gathering dust, unlikely to ever be seen by the scientific community. Was I interested? I was.

I was shown to the most astonishing office. Its window overlooked lush green trees, but the room was dark; the room was piled floor-to-ceiling with dust-covered papers. The only open space on the desk was about two feet square. Even the desk chair was covered with papers. "You happy?" Barbara asked me. "Yes," I replied and got to work on the Ivory Coast data.

Hundreds of community health workers in the Ivory Coast had been specifically trained to follow a person (man, woman or child) around for seven days and write down a numeric code for every activity the person did. The data had been gathered for 3,352 people from four communities, 1,787 women and 1,565 men. It was a unique analysis as to how an ancient culture, where people lived an agricultural way of life with little use of machines, influenced people's activities. Data were compiled for the 22,397 person-days and 23 million data points. For all age ranges, we found that women worked three hours a day more than men.[13] Men had more chair-based relaxation time and leisure-associated travel (e.g., time to go to the bar).

Meticulous data documented all the tasks that women and men performed. Women conducted about a quarter of the agricultural work, such as bundling up crops and hand-carrying them on their heads to market. In addition to this, they conducted *all* domestic tasks, including carrying wood and water into the home and hand-milling flour. Men worked exclusively on agricultural tasks, particularly seeding, scything and banging posts into the ground. Men were the sole scythe users because their physique lends itself to longer arm sweeps and greater cutting efficiency.[14] Only men bang posts into the ground, however, because these posts demarcate land ownership, and in these cultures, women cannot own land.

The overall analysis demonstrated that the cultural norms in this society resulted in women having far greater calorie needs than had ever been thought before. In fact, World Food Bank equations underestimated these women's calorie needs by a third! What was worse was that the culture also defined who got to eat first. There was a distinct pecking order when food was put on the table; men and boys ate first, then the women.[15]

Here you see the power of culture. Not only did the culture drive up the work burden and calorie needs of the women; it also disadvantaged them from getting food. As a result, when the crops failed and food was scarce, women starved.

Whether you have an unused mini-gym in the office next to your desk or you are in an agricultural community in the Ivory Coast, culture is a major driver of your activity level and access to chairs.

To release corporations from lethal sitting, we needed to define a new culture of work.

OFFICE OF THE FUTURE

One day in 2007 my assistant, Amy Flickinger, telephoned me. "Dr. Levine, I have John Folkestad on the line. He insists that he talk with you." My knee-jerk response was to decline. "But," Amy protested, "it's the fifth time he's called today." I remembered how I felt when Professor Fartoobusy ignored me, and I took the call.

John Folkestad was cofounder of a midsize, highly successful financial services business in Minneapolis called Salo. He asked if

I would come and give a talk to his staff about NEAT and lethal sitting. I explained that I simply didn't have the time.

Two weeks later, after being repeatedly called by John, I walked into Salo's offices in downtown Minneapolis, 100 miles from the lab. Salo was housed in a converted warehouse, redesigned with modern lines and bright colors. In less than a minute, John burst through the office doors to meet me, words pouring out. No introductions. "Dr. Levine, I love, love, love what you're doing, you've got to do it here at Salo and you've got to do it here first. I'm your first volunteer. You know what a six-pack is? I've got a keg." Amy Langer, a trim brunette with a giant smile, joined us. She explained that she and John were the joint founders of Salo, and they wanted, more than anything, for their employees to have the opportunity to work healthily. "After the twins," she went on, and patted her tummy, "I've got a few baby pounds to lose." John interrupted. "I think it's great business too," he added.

"Why don't we walk and talk about it?" I said. John bounded out of the office; Amy and I followed. It was winter; we started to walk through the sky bridges that connect Minneapolis office buildings. John's enthusiasm was like a fast-replicating virus—completely unstoppable. Every time Amy tried to interject calm, John simply took a breath and spoke in torrents about his need to have Salo lead the world in this new NEAT chair-free revolution. We came to a large escalator going up. Amy stepped on and I followed. Much to my astonishment, John took the down-going escalator and sprinted up it against the flow. More astonishing still, he continued to talk to me as he did so.

John's passion was a force of nature. Amy's calm was an island of safety. I understood why Salo was so successful. "Doctor, we'll do whatever you tell us," John said. I smiled, extended my hand and said, "Can't wait to work with you."

I wanted to transform Salo, not only into the first NEAT chair-restricted office in the world but also into my new lab. I told John and Amy what I had in mind. "I want to build a laboratory right inside of your offices so we can test whether our chair-escape programs work in a real office environment." Amy was silent; then she spoke. "Surely a laboratory has to be in a research institute." I explained that that is normally so, but I wanted to measure how real people, in a real work environment, respond to the new NEAT chair-free work style. To do so, I needed a lab on site rather than bringing subjects to our lab 100 miles away. There was silence.

"Great!" John said finally. "We can give you the massage room, and you can convert it into a lab." I have never worked for an organization that has an in-office massage room. Perhaps finance management was not as dull as I had thought.

If science is to be valuable in society, it has to measure people where they are: at work, play and home. The idea of creating laboratories in carved-out public spaces intrigued me. By embedding a laboratory in a corporation, I could work out how to reverse the chair sentence where people live their day-to-day lives. I figured if we could build a laboratory in one corporation, we could do it in 100. Public laboratories could be built in schools, old-age homes and unemployment offices. Could disused post offices become community labs? To understand what works for real people, we have to conduct science where people live their lives.

It seemed like a good idea, but building a lab inside a corporate office is rather like driving a car on the ocean—it's just not done. And so, in order to deliver on this audacious plan, I needed an audacious planner. I advertised for someone who wanted to change the world. Hundreds of resumes came in.

I interviewed people with decades of experience. When I explained that I wanted to start to build labs in offices, schools and communities, several applicants laughed, and many withdrew their applications. The second-to-last interview was with a young man who had lost his job due to downsizing. He showed up five minutes late, wearing an open-necked shirt and jeans. "Let's get this one over," I thought, and I told the man his interview would be short. "Why don't we walk and talk?" Gabe Koepp suggested.

I asked Gabe about his background, and he told me that he had trained in exercise science, had been a wrestling coach and a contractor, had run an obesity task force and was currently getting his MBA online. His accomplishments were remarkable for a 30-year-old, but as he spoke the cadence of his voice barely changed. It was as if he were reciting a shopping list.

Gabe had far less laboratory experience than all of the other applicants. I told him what I had in mind: "I want to build scientific laboratories where people live their lives," I said. He asked, "You mean like in schools and offices?" I nodded. He shrugged. "That should not be a problem," he said, and then he was silent. His interview lasted less than ten minutes. It did not cross my mind to ask Gabe how he would actually achieve this, but six weeks later he had.

Gabe borrowed equipment, found local collaborators and usurped resources. He constructed a fully functioning laboratory inside Salo, better than 95 percent of other labs in the United States. Equipment aside, we needed a strategy—a plan—to orchestrate the release of Salo's workers from their chairs.

We developed the plan in 12 layers.

Layer 1. Culture and Leadership

John and Amy not only gave us a carte blanche to transform their company's practice, they brought in everyone, from senior management to the janitorial team. Salo would be corporate health pioneers. The culture shift had begun.

Layer 2. Systems and Procedures— Get Everyone's Buy-in

We asked Salo to list its critical operational systems. We worked with Salo's information technology team, healthcare provider, workflow managers, productivity teams, secretarial pool, attorneys, janitorial staff and phone providers. We also worked with the heating/air-conditioning company to ensure that the space would remain in thermal comfort and the electricity providers to ensure that power points could be moved at will. We developed a detailed procedural plan and an intricate floor map to ensure that the company's systems and procedures continued to function effectively, but in a way that facilitated NEAT and allowed chairs to be set aside.

Gabe hired a dynamic woman named Desiree Ahrens, whose new company provided health coaches. Desiree let us establish the training procedures, and Salo allowed us five minutes of coaching time per employee per day. With Desiree's team on board, we had therapeutic hands on the office floor.

Layer 3. Physical Infrastructure

A local architectural firm wanted to enter the active-work business as part of its own strategic plan. It developed a physical infrastructure plan so that a walking track now circled the office, Ping-Pong and gaming tables could be moved in (John and Amy paid for those) and chairs became architectural accents rather than the dominant furnishing.

Layer 4. Furnishings

Two dozen treadmill desks were moved in, and a dozen desks and chairs were removed. Some desks were lengthened to allow mixed working—treadmill plus chair. We changed artwork to pieces that showed people being active and happy.

Layer 5. Biotech Self-Monitoring

We completed a technology build using a new company we had developed so that each employee received their own MEMS chip accelerometer device, which we called Gruve®, that clocked every movement and all inactivity.

Layer 6. Develop Personal Plans Using the Five Weapons

We developed comprehensive, 12-week written plans for all the employees. The plans did not just involve lethal sitting but also stress, sleep, eating and what we called the dream tunnel: where everyone got to spell out their dream and develop a plan on how to achieve it. We pushed the five weapons of behavioral change remorselessly: stimulus control, monitoring, cognitive reconstruction, reward/penalty systems and social support.

Layer 7. Enhance the Group Dynamic

Every Monday I gave a lethal sitting seminar to the whole company—all of whom stood. On Wednesday there was a Salo-led educational activity. On Friday there was a group nutritional activity that incorporated a discussion, led by the employees, about active ideas for the weekend. The whole company participated.

Layer 8. Science Is Power

Gabe's office-based laboratory came to fruition. In the office, we could measure how much body fat people had, how many calories they burned sitting at traditional desks or while having a walk-and-talk meeting. We measured blood sugar and cholesterol, and we completed intricate isotope measurements to validate the new Gruve devices. We brought in a famed economics team to independently analyze the company's productivity and healthcare costs.

Contrary to what we expected, the employees loved the lab. I still remember one man whose eyes came alive when we showed him that his calorie burn increased by 210 calories/hour when he walked at 1.5 mph during a walking meeting.

The lab enabled us to directly measure what components of the office transformation worked for which employees, and to what benefit.

Layer 9. Test, Test Again and Retest

Every part of the plan was tested and retested. We ran dummy runs on weekends and had up to three contingency plans for some of the trickier components. Maybe we overplanned, but that was better than collapsing.

Layer 10. Oversight and Ethics

We had an oversight board that included employees at all levels who advised us and helped us continuously tweak the program. It allowed problems to be voiced from Salo (without John and Amy in the room) and from us. We also had a physician on call to deal with any health complaints or issues. The Mayo Clinic Ethics Committee approved every piece of our plan, in particular, how workers' data and identities would be protected.

Layer 11. Mission

It is critical to convey a mission not only at the start but throughout a deployment. The entire company, and ourselves, had a unifying mission: Our shared goal was to bring health and happiness to every employee at Salo. We knew mistakes would be made and challenges would have to be overcome, but throughout the entire process, we also knew that our shared ethic was pure and powerful. Together, we wanted to free Salo employees from their chair sentence and help them reach their personal dreams and have fabulous health.

Layer 12. Sustain for Two Years

It is great to start a program enthusiastically, but if it cannot be sustained at two years, it has less benefit. So-called sustainability plans actually evolve over time, but unless you can conjecture how a program will be sustained, there is a fundamental fault.

Why two years? People cannot think in infinitesimal time spans, and the data suggest that health changes sustained at two years have the possibility of long-term benefit.[16]

As weeks became months, Salo workers crept out of their chairs and onto the walking tracks, step devices and treadmill desks. The entire atmosphere of the office changed. On one occasion, I went to Salo straight from a long flight from London. As I walked in, Amy was walking around the office walking track, marked with pink duct tape. Beside her walked a colleague who was significantly heavier. They were in intense discussion. Both wore their regular work clothes, both were working. There was no way that these two individuals would have exercised together, but here they were, active, working and productive.

We could hardly believe the data coming in from our onsite lab. Not only was weight declining, but so too was body fat, blood sugar and cholesterol values; the health numbers improved week after week. Also, as body fat was declining, muscle mass was increasing. The financial analysis, however, provided the greatest surprise. When the financial analysis was calculated, not only had productivity improved by 15 percent, but the company also showed its best quarter profits ever. NEAT work was profitable; improved health was a side effect.

John and Amy, the cofounders, were ecstatic. "When this chair-escape program began," Amy explained, "the office staff had a certain monotonous work routine that you could feel the moment you walked in. Once the NEAT program had begun and the people started using the treadmill desks and the walking paths, a whole stack of other activities followed." Employees started a competition for healthy snacks at work, she explained. The results were so tasty that it became an unwritten policy to stop bringing in cake and share homemade health snacks instead. People started to take the NEAT philosophy home. One family, instead of having a pizza party, had a tobogganing party. Amy said there were unexpected changes in individuals and how she interacted with them. She found staff members to be more self-confident and to take on challenges they hadn't normally taken on before. This happened not only at work but at home as well. John added, "It is easy to explain why the company did so well since you guys came. Everyone just has been happier." Multiple studies show that happy employees are more productive and more innovative.[17]

The story of Salo spread like wildfire, and national television came knocking at their door. ABC News' *20/20* ran a feature on August 1, 2008, and the office of the future was now the NEAT chairless office of the present. Gabe's phone began to ring off the hook. More than five years later, Salo's chair-escape program continues. Weight loss company-wide averages 9 pounds per person per year and profitability has continued to increase.[18] The culture at Salo has been redefined to what they call "a culture of movement."

By the end of the Salo project, our lab capability had expanded: We had developed sensing technologies, NEAT furniture (not only did we have treadmill desks; Ergotron released a range of inexpensive standing desks), comprehensive personalized chair-escape plans, the necessary systems and procedures and detailed validation data—we had an arsenal to end lethal sitting.

We had learned that people can get an extra 2 hours and 15 minutes a day of walking *while at work*. We discovered that after corporate chair release, productivity and profit improve alongside employee happiness and better health.

With this advanced capability, we started to deploy NEAT programs across dozens of corporations but always with the 12-layered strategy we'd developed at Salo.

THE 12 LAYERS OF DEPLOYMENT

Layer 1. Culture and Leadership.
Layer 2. Systems and Procedures—Get Everyone's
    Buy-in.
Layer 3. Physical Infrastructure.

Layer 4. Furnishings.

Layer 5. Biotech Self-Monitoring.

Layer 6. Develop Personal Plans Using the Five Weapons of Behavioral Change.

Layer 7. Enhance the Group Dynamic.

Layer 8. Science Is Power.

Layer 9. Test, Test Again and Retest.

Layer 10. Oversight and Ethics.

Layer 11. Mission.

Layer 12. Sustain for Two Years.

BOTTOM-LINE BENEFIT

Workplace NEAT programs offer eight consistent benefits[19]:

1. Increased productivity.
2. Improved health measures and decreased healthcare costs.
3. Decreased employee stress.
4. The ripple effect: Although these programs are delivered to the workplace, we consistently see the benefits ripple into employee's home lives.
5. Increased happiness.
6. Positive atmosphere.
7. Decreased staff turnover.
8. Hiring advantage.

Walk into a NEAT office, where people have put aside their chairs, and you will sense the electricity of humans living as we were designed to live.

NEAT workplaces attract talent. Young talent is not drawn to a company only by salary because salary levels are fairly standard for most job descriptions. The best and brightest come to a company because they have a good feel for the firm. Imagine being a young financial hotshot with several offers on the table. Would you choose a company where the culture is so intense that you cannot even go to a mini-gym in the room next door? Or would you chose Salo, where you move all day, play pool at lunchtime, work in a culture of dynamic fun, where minor disputes are solved with rock-paper-scissors, where the woman at her standing desk across the office is performing a jazz concert this weekend and the guy at treadmill desk 8 just wrote his first novel? In NEAT offices, everyone is included, all employees share a mission and people are happier and healthier.

The verdict is in; chair-based work is harmful for health, happiness and profitability. Change must occur. Corporate America needs to collectively get up. I foresee office environments where being up, moving, dynamic, happy and productive is the *default*. In these forward-thinking corporations, people will be up and moving throughout the day, and they will take chair breaks from time to time and occasional naps—this is how our bodies are designed to function. Work needs to be NEAT overhauled, not only to enable employees to survive but to maximize the innate human drive to be creative and productive. The new *default* is up!

QUIZ: OFFICE OLYMPICS

Here are some activities for the office. Which one is associated with worse health and lowest productivity?

1. Ban email for certain time periods (e.g., "No email from 2 to 5 p.m. on Wednesday.")
2. Stand up and pace when talking on the phone.
3. Have small, low-cost stepping devices in the conference room.
4. Move your chair elsewhere to make you consider standing while at work.
5. Use a treadmill desk.
6. Sit on a stabilizer ball.

7. Encourage people to socialize at work and to laugh.
8. Provide free MP3 players for employees to take a musical stroll.
9. Link healthcare plans to the amount of daily movement employees complete.
10. Take a five- to ten-minute walking break each hour.
11. Encourage people to reach for their aspirations.
12. Hold walk-and-talk meetings.
13. Let company art gallery outings replace all-you-can-eat specials.
14. Mark walking trails with tape on the office floor.
15. Create an office guide to nearby outdoor trails.
16. Use social media to encourage active lunches.
17. Move trash cans and printers to increase office walking.
18. Provide desk-exercise equipment (e.g., hand weights).
19. Have an office dog.
20. Encourage afternoon naps.
21. Do arm curls with a ream of paper.
22. Do knee bends at your chair.
23. Perform ten push-ups after every sale.
24. Establish reward programs for increased NEAT.
25. Hang a pet photo competition in the office stairwell.
26. Sit motionless in a chair for eight hours a day.

Sitting in a chair for eight hours a day is the last thing you want if you desire a productive, happy and healthy workforce.

12

LEARN!

Education Solutions

AS A CHILD, MY TEACHERS CASTIGATED ME FOR FIDGETING during lessons. How strange it was, 30 years later, to return to school with a mandate to encourage children to move not only during recess and at home but even during their lessons.

In 2006, the NEAT lab was working with a federal agency to deploy a NEAT-based workplace program that included the 12 layers of deployment (described in chapter 11) when my long-suffering assistant, Amy, received another phone call. I was on my office treadmill, reading some poems by Robert Frost when my pager went off. Immediately I heard the anxiety in Amy's voice. "Dr. Levine, you have to take this call . . . now!" When I did, a woman's voice said, "Dr. Levine, I work with . . ." I almost dropped the phone. The call was from the White House.

I was asked a simple question. If sitting is so bad for workers and NEAT-active work has so many benefits for employee health and productivity, surely this must also be the case for children. "What are you doing for kids?" I was asked. At the time, childhood obesity was looming in the scientific community as an impending health disaster, but its importance had not yet attracted public attention. I hung up the phone, not quite sure what to do. I left the hospital and went for a walk in the park.

IF YOU NEED SOMETHING DONE, FIND PEOPLE WHO ARE BUSY

I went to talk to Shelly and Gabe and asked how we could adapt our corporate strategies for schools. Normally when you explain to your team that you want them to double their workload, you expect a little pushback. Shelly bounced out of her chair and said, "When can we begin?" Gabe smiled confidently and said, "Let's just get out and do this."

A week later we advertised for a new faculty member. Several young scientists responded, but none caught my interest until I saw the resume of Lorraine Lanningham-Foster. Lorraine had been well trained in animal science, but it was the letter she wrote that impressed me. There was strength in her words. It is funny how small things can affect you, but as soon as I read this letter I knew she was the one.

I invited her for an interview. It just so happened that when we were booking the tickets, I was in Amy's office. She said to me, "The ticket is $560. But first class is $610." I said, "Book the first-class ticket."

Lorraine came to Mayo Clinic in Rochester. She was from Florida and had a gentle smile and a cutting sense of humor; I liked her immediately. Lorraine's resume was not impressive, but her manner was as much maternal as ruthlessly professional. It transpired that she had been offered a job at another premier obesity research facility. Upon hearing that, I hung my head and said good-bye.

A few weeks later Lorraine called. "I want to come to the NEAT lab, at Mayo," she said.

I asked her why she had chosen Mayo over the other research center. She laughed. "You guys bought me a first-class ticket.

Anyone who treats an interviewee that well is going to look after my professional development." And so with Lorraine at the helm, we began to cross-train our corporate programs for schools. From the Salo experience, I realized that we needed to have a demonstration project. We needed to reinvent school.

REINVENTING SCHOOL

Everybody has an opinion about schools, so we convened a conference of 100 teachers to discuss the idea of the NEAT-active schooling. We ended up with 114 ideas along with 54 barriers to implementing the NEAT mandate—everything from janitorial issues to liability. However, it was clear that teachers were passionately seeking health solutions for their students. The fear that teachers expressed most often concerned the demands on their time. With all the state and federal test reporting they had to do, they had little time left to decrease chair time and encourage NEAT in the classroom; educational scores were key. Also, we discovered that as schools worked through funding shortfalls, physical education teachers were the first to be let go, recess had become shorter—20 minutes over the course of the day for some children—and classrooms were frequently too full. In the United States, only 4 percent of elementary schools, 8 percent of middle schools and 2 percent of high schools provide daily physical education.[1] We were also told that many fidgety children (probably those with high NEAT in their brain circuits) were frequently medicated for attention-deficit/hyperactivity disorder (ADHD). The teachers had abundant passion for change, but no resources, time or know-how as to how to do it.

It struck me, though, that the input we had gleaned was not from the perspective of the customer—the students. I was a child who spent most of his school time staring out of windows, sleeping and firing paper pellets at my friends; I wondered what kids would say about NEAT chair-free learning.

The most enthusiastic teacher in our 100-teacher conference was Phil Rynearson. I telephoned him and asked if I could come and speak to his students. Two days later Lorraine and I held focus groups with his class. Phil went a step further; after our session, he gave his fourth and fifth grade students a homework assignment to come up with suggestions on how to build the perfect NEAT-active school. Lorraine and I returned a week later to review their ideas.

The children immediately understood the concept of NEAT and the poison of the chair. Their ideas were mind blowing! For example, one boy had the idea of learning in a hot tub so that he could play in the snow in between lessons. His idea was to have a hot tub that did not contain water but instead a dry heated substance. I thought that the idea of a hot tub that doesn't get you wet was brilliant. Out of curiosity, I went to the US patent web portal; six weeks before the assignment, a patent had been filed for a hot tub filled with heated ceramic beads funded by the army, whereby soldiers could get heat therapy for strained muscles but not get wet.

One girl had the idea of a robust standing desk on wheels. It was designed to create a private space for students to work in. I liked the design so much I called up a friend at a school furniture manufacturer, which started to build prototypes.

Idea by idea, the students reinvented not only the classroom but the school. The overriding concept was that they wanted a learning village they could stroll around in during the school day. They wanted it built so that the different parts of the village had different functions: shaded areas for quiet study, open areas for collaborative work and spaces for sports. They liked the idea of openness and bright light so they could see nature outside and the gardens they planted.

As for the classroom, since these kids were from Minnesota, their choice of classroom design was an ice hockey arena. Obviously learning on ice wasn't practical, but there is an ice-hard plastic flooring material that is almost as good as ice and does not require freezing.

The kids designed the entire school space, the classroom and all the components in it. They also discussed with us the need for educational software and iPods that would make NEAT learning dynamic. They envisioned artwork that would be suspended from the ceilings but would need to be replaced frequently to keep it fresh. They had ideas about the cafeteria, but interestingly, for as many spontaneous ideas they had about NEAT dynamic learning, they provided few food changes; nachos and pizza were still at the top of their list. Also, the kids did not discuss classroom behavior, attentiveness or grades, which had been the focal points at the teachers' conference.

FROM DREAM TO REALITY: THE SCHOOL OF THE FUTURE

As we were developing the NEAT school concept, I happened to be a volunteer on the local school board. I wrote an advisory document for the board about active learning; the first half contained the wish list and concerns from the 100-teacher conference; the second half of the document was the students' solutions. The board asked me to give a presentation, which I did late one Thursday evening. I anticipated uproarious laughter and cynical smiles. What blew me away were the words of the superintendent of schools, who was in his last year of a 20-year tenure. He stood up and said, "We need to identify one school and try this NEAT learning." The motion was unanimously approved.

One of the school board members, Wes Emmert, came up to talk with me. We spoke for an hour. He explained that he was from the Rochester Athletic Club, which had just built a new 6,000-square-foot annex that it didn't quite know what to do with. Could I create the School of the Future there? I smiled at Wes. "You bet!"

The next morning I went up to the Rochester Athletic Club and met with Wes and his boss, Greg Lappin, and I showed them the children's NEAT School of the Future drawings. "Beautiful," Greg said. "We have to finish the space anyway. Why don't we build what the kids want?" It was as simple as that! Over the next four months, the Rochester Athletic Club built the School of the Future based on the dreams of the children.

It was an easy decision for the school superintendent to assign Phil Rynearson's fourth and fifth grade classroom at Elton Hills Elementary School as the test bed for this new adventure. Phil walked through the cavernous School of the Future as it was being built. I thought he would be wowed, but his focus was on teaching kids. Phil told me that he needed acoustic equipment so that the teacher's voice could be heard as the kids moved around. He needed to test the technology and educational computer suite to ensure that it worked the way he needed. The technology build Phil demanded would cost about $350,000. He said, "Unless I can teach my kids properly, we're not coming." Phil was just like some of the hardnosed CEOs I'd worked with, but his goal was the education of his kids. I began to panic; what Phil wanted was unprecedented.

At that time I was scheduled to go to Jamaica and work on our program where we were investigating NEAT levels in people working in agricultural communities. I almost canceled, but I needed to get away, so off I went to see Professor Terrence Forrester in Kingston. We had dinner, and Terrence could see I was distraught. "I don't know how I'm going to pull off this active School of the Future," I told him. He said, "There's someone you need to meet."

Terrence took me to a school in Spanish Town, 15 miles west of Kingston. "Tell Chloe what you are trying to do," he said. While having a cup of tea, I told Chloe, the head teacher, about our redesigned NEAT School of the Future in Rochester. She burst out laughing and said, "Come with me." Her class of ten-year-olds had assembled for an English lesson. Chloe took

the kids to the playground and gave them a word to spell—
"caterpillar." As they spelled out each letter, they hopped on
one leg. She then had them spell another word followed by another. After about a dozen words, the children were sweating
and smiling and she called out to them, "Good spellers." I got
the point.

In Rochester, the School of the Future had already cost almost a quarter million dollars when the building and refurbish-
ment costs were totted up, but all it really took was the will of the
teacher and a group of hopping, happy children (Layer 1: Culture!). The whole day was like this; the children danced around
in a circle as they recited poetry and did running races after each
times table. When Terrence told Chloe it was my birthday, I was
allowed to join in the running races. At the end of the school day,
I watched the children leave (on foot) and thanked Chloe. She
smiled and raised an eyebrow above sparkling brown eyes. "They
learn so well, and my students still have to walk an hour just to
get home. Keep on with your project," she said.

So much has changed in the United States; in 1969 42 percent of school-aged children biked or walked to school, compared
with 16 percent in 2001[2]; our children, like their parents, have
become chair sentenced. I realized right then that if we could
change the culture of American schools, we could win. The
School of the Future was not the end product but the starting
point.

Back in my hotel that night, I thought about the insanity of
a new generation of unhealthy American children. There is an
expectation of poor health in the modern child; pharmaceutical companies are rubbing their hands with glee that every child
will get a polypill at school to prevent diabetes and high blood
pressure just like I used to get school milk.[3] Putting cholesterol-
lowering medications into the water supply even has been suggested.[4] And it isn't just America; half of children in Beijing have
obesity,[5] obesity is accelerating faster than car sales in India, and
in several Arabic-speaking countries, most children already have

obesity.[6] Unless we get up and act, my grandchildren will never know what a healthy, unmedicated person looks like.

Late that night I wrote an email to Tony Fadell at Apple, explaining the monstrous school project we had started and how we would need $350,000 worth of technological solutions. That night I didn't sleep well. I had bizarre dreams about children dancing in vats of mud. The faster they danced, the quicker they sank. In the morning, I saw that Tony had replied. "I have spoken to John Couch, our vice president for education at Apple, and he wants to meet with you tomorrow at 9 a.m."

I said good-bye to Terrence over breakfast and changed my flights to take me to San Francisco in the afternoon. The following morning, at 8 a.m., I walked into the foyer of Apple Computer. At 9:15, I politely reminded the receptionist that I was waiting. A quarter of an hour later, a tall, young, mega-trendy, super-slim man rushed down the stairs toward me. "You are Dr. Levine?" he said. "We were expecting you yesterday." (I'd failed to notice that Tony had replied instantly to email. My appointment with John Couch had been the morning before!)

"All I need is five minutes," I told the assistant. "I've come from Jamaica," I added. He looked me up and down. "Okay, Mr. Couch will see you at 10. But he'll be between meetings. He'll barely have five minutes."

I was shown to a large conference room. I had prepared a 45-minute PowerPoint presentation, which I ditched. My heart thumped hard as I waited. John Couch burst into the room followed by the tall, lanky assistant. "Welcome, Dr. Levine. I am so sorry that I don't have as much time with you as I wanted. What can I do for you?"

I pitched the School of the Future in less than a minute; I explained that I had collaborated with a group of kids and redesigned the school system to promote NEAT. I told him what they wanted was a village-like atmosphere where they could move around freely and learn. That took 30 seconds. "The trouble is," I explained, "we need a complete sound and computer solution to enable the kids to learn as they are moving around this space." That took another 30 seconds. John turned to his assistant and said, "Give them what they need." Then he walked out, followed two feet behind by his assistant. I had spent 20 hours getting to this meeting, which had lasted less than two minutes, but I had achieved what I needed.

I packed up my computer and was about to leave the conference room when the door burst open again. John walked in, with Steve Jobs behind. "Tell Steve what you told me," he said. I gave Mr. Jobs the eight-second version. "Great idea," the master said, and left.

Two weeks later, three shipping crates arrived at the School of the Future from Cupertino, the home of Apple Computer, along with two technicians (no, not inside the crates). The School of the Future already looked like a village, complete with sitting area, café, classrooms that looked like hockey arenas and basketball courts. The Apple technicians worked round the clock for three days, and by the time they were done, we had a fully functional and tested education suite ready to run. I invited Phil Rynearson for a demonstration.

Phil walked in, looking skeptical from the get-go. We showed him the teaching suite: Every pupil would get a laptop and iPod (iPads had not been invented yet). Phil would have a giant console that allowed him remote access to any of the students' computers. In this way he could review a pupil's work in real time and start a chat, with audio, video or text, wherever the student was in the futuristic space. In addition, filming software enabled the students to record their questions and prepare video presentations. We also had concert-style acoustics with noise cancellation so that the teacher's voice could be heard wherever students might be. The demo took an hour. Phil looked at me. "Dr. Levine, this project is going to change the world," he said. I thought of Chloe's happy, active learners. "Your kids designed this," I said.

And so the School of the Future was complete. The building looked incredible, like a miniature, pristine town center. We visited the students in their existing classroom and gave each girl and boy their allocated computer and iPod. The students instantaneously worked out how to access all of the capabilities before Phil even began to explain. Kids have an incredible capacity to adopt technological solutions far faster than adults.

Two weeks before the School of the Future opened, Lorraine, Chinmay, Shelly and I went down to the regular school and taped sensors to the legs and backs of the students. We wanted to measure their sitting and NEAT activity levels at baseline in the traditional school environment before they moved to the School of the Future.

DAY ONE OF THE FUTURE

The day of the School of the Future's opening came fast. We tested everything (Layer 9); we were ready. Despite eight inches of snow, all the major TV networks came to Rochester to meet Phil's kids on their first day in the School of the Future.

I sat with the kids on the school bus as we drove to their dream school. Their excitement was tangible. They chatted and jumped up and down on the seats. It was contagious. Teacher Phil came to the front of the bus and told the kids to simmer down. The 13-year-old boy sitting beside me frowned. All of a sudden I was 30 years younger; I stopped bouncing and sat still.

Very few children can say that they have designed their own school and have been greeted at school by truckloads of media. These children could! The kids ignored the television cameras and ran into their new school. The school superintendent had allowed Phil and his students two days purely to acclimate to the new facility. But as I mentioned, children are adept at adapting. Within an hour Phil had them strolling around their new classroom, a hockey arena. The floor was rigid plastic. There were large rubber benches so that the kids could take chair breaks if they wanted to. There were hockey goal nets too; kids love to learn in forts.

Phil introduced the students to the specially designed school furniture. Each student had a portable desk that resembled a preacher's lectern and a portable whiteboard about three feet high by one and a half feet wide. This was the student's personal whiteboard, which was so lightweight (about a pound) that it could be carried around. Sweeping his long arms into the air, Phil explained the need for sound control and demoed the acoustic system, which resembled a rock concert system. There were several small standing cubicles on wheels for more private work—cubicles designed by one of the students.

Next Phil asked the students what they all thought of the space. One boy raised his hand. "We are pioneers," he said. The students understood that somehow a new type of education that *embraced* health needed to be devised. By then I had delivered programs to more than 60 corporations, but never before had I heard a more profound understanding of the need of change. Phil then explained to the students that the superintendent had allowed two full days just to get accustomed to the new school. He shrugged his shoulders and said that it looked as if the students already had gotten the idea. The kids nodded, and Phil began to teach; they had been there less than two hours.

NEW SCHOOL ENVIRONMENT:
LESSONS LEARNED

I went to the School of the Future every day for weeks: sometimes for 20 minutes, sometimes for a few hours, just to watch how the children responded. I carefully watched the teachers too. I wanted to see how they overcame the barriers and challenges that NEAT schooling raised.

The kids ambled around the space and moved desks and laptops with them, as if they had always gone to this school. Given the chance, kids move—but they also rest. For instance, in the "skating arena" classroom, kids might be standing at their desks, walking around or actually sitting on the rubber benches.

Without warning, a sitter might stand and stander might sit. Kids popped up and down, walked hither and thither, without obvious pattern. From what Phil told me, the kids seemed to be learning well, but we would not know until the end-of-year standardized tests.

After two months we sent out an electronic survey that asked the students what they thought of the School of the Future. The most common word in their responses was "Love."

The teachers, as a group, admitted that they had been somewhat skeptical about the school but had participated predominantly because of their respect for Phil. They reported that they found the students to be more ready to learn. Phil put it this way:

> I noticed several major changes in my students. There was less movement for movement's sake—fewer trips to the bathroom or water fountain. Students shifted their bodies and changed positions when they needed to in order to stay focused. And students were able to move themselves away from other students who might be distracting or bothering them. This led to much less bickering and fewer distractions from classwork.

Despite the technological challenges, the teachers found it easier and more pleasurable to teach in the School of the Future. In fact, a number of teachers who had not participated in the project contacted me about doing so.

The most interesting responses, however, were from the parents. They reported that their children came home from school more relaxed and happier to do homework. Several reports stated that the children couldn't wait to get to school in the morning and would have stayed longer at school if possible. Many parents reported that their kids were happier and even that their own relationships with their children had improved. Several parents told us that they had started their own health and fitness programs inspired by their children, and we received numerous reports of parents changing home nutrition to healthier options and converting chair-based weekends to active ones.

One of the most inspiring reports we received was about a girl I will refer to as Michelle (it is not her real name); she had a diagnosis of ADHD and was on Ritalin. Before the School of the Future, Phil told me that Michelle had to be excused every half hour to go to the toilet. The girl's English comprehension and mathematical skills had fallen far behind state standards. The change seen in Michelle in the School of the Future was impressive. The first thing that Phil noticed was that the girl no longer took half-hourly bathroom breaks; she had been one of the most distracted students during lessons because of the ADHD. In week 5, the music teacher excitedly showed Phil the composition Michelle had composed on her computer. Not only was the music well scripted, but the lyrics were beautiful. Michelle's composition was the best in the class. The girl's spelling improved too; Phil had Michelle learn the week's spelling words letter by letter while throwing balls through the basketball hoop. Mathematics was next. Michelle literally made a 180-degree turn. By the time the school year finished, Michelle had caught up completely. Phil told me, "She is easily averaging a B+." Two weeks later, Michelle's medications were stopped. The note of thanks I received from the girl's father almost brought me to tears.

What troubles me is this: How many more Michelles are needlessly on ADHD medication and not reaching their potential? After the publicity the School of the Future received in 2007, I have been approached by numerous educators troubled by children misdiagnosed as having ADHD. Several programs have already begun providing children with ADHD ball chairs or treadmills or simply permitting them to stroll around the classroom during lessons. According to the Centers for Disease Control, 5 million children in the United States have been diagnosed with ADHD; that is about one in ten kids aged 3 to

17.[7] Wouldn't it be a tragedy if even a quarter of these diagnoses (more than 1 million children) were purely a consequence of the chair sentence—and could be helped just by reversing it?

Once the children had been working in the School of the Future for several months, we repeated the measurements of NEAT activity using our MEMS (micro electro-mechanical systems) accelerometer sensors. The children's activity levels had *doubled* compared to their levels in the traditional chair-based classroom. In fact, these children moved as much as when they were on summer vacation. (We measured them during their vacations too.) In other words, it seemed as if the School of the Future enabled children to move naturally, the way their bodies were designed to move.

When state educational scores came in, the scores of students in the School of the Future had improved by 10 to 20 percent above their benchmark.[8] Since those results and others were published, it has become irrefutable that active learning is associated with improved educational attainment and better health. Many schools in a number of countries got the message. Over the last decade, NEAT-active schooling has taken off in Germany, the United Kingdom, Sweden and Australia.

Interest started to grow in the United States as well; however, the US challenges were great because teachers were overwhelmed with governmental requirements for student testing, recess time was shrinking and physical education teachers were being let go. These and other factors sapped teachers' energies for taking on large new programs, although NEAT-active, chairless classrooms cropped up from time to time, most often led by grassroots initiatives and federal grants.

One example was in Idaho Falls, where a mother became so concerned about the health of her son in middle school that she single-handedly gained approval from the school board and classroom teachers to enact a NEAT school program—complete with standing desks. She raised the funds from local businesses.

It was worth her effort; sitting time decreased, and educational scores and classroom behavior improved.[9]

SUSTAINABLE ACTIVE SCHOOLING

Seeing the success of these NEAT school programs, I became interested in how sustainable models of active schooling could be supported.

I like the idea of *complete* school redesign because the notion of active learning requires buy-in not only from students—who immediately take to it—but also teachers, parents, principals, school boards, janitorial staff and ultimately school builders. In a Colorado school I visited, children have aspirations to join the Olympic ski team. They complete their lessons in the morning and ski in the afternoon. This model also is deployed in London at the Royal School of Ballet, where the school day is basically divided into two: learning lessons half of the day and sports/dance for the rest of the day. These students have high educational attainment and are high achievers in their selected activity, whether it's skiing or ballet. On the face of it, this approach seems extreme, but it proves that high-quality, high-intensity education leaves substantial portions of the school day available for physical activity. Children in the sports schools are healthy and well educated and have a shot at their dreams. Why don't all children?

Another comprehensive model is MindStream Academy in Hilton Head, South Carolina, a boarding school dedicated to children with severe obesity. Ray Travaglione, who earned his educational stripes running a school for child golf prodigies, leads MindStream. He is dynamic and he believes in what he is doing. The school is set on a 43-acre horse ranch in beautiful surroundings; one of the on-site sports offered is horseback riding. All the students are teens challenged with substantial excess body weight; some have diabetes, asthma and hypertension, and most have been bullied because of their weight.

Although the semester price is a hefty $28,500, children from less well-off backgrounds can attend on scholarships. Children here lose about 100 pounds over a six-month period, although the long-term outcomes are unknown. This is an immersion system whereby children live health rather than being taught it. At MindStream, healthy learning and nutritious eating (much of the produce is grown on the school grounds) are norms.

What impressed me most, however, was the social support the students offered each other. I attended a group meeting of 16 students, all of whom had lost 80 to 110 pounds. I listened and was moved by how they interacted; the mutual support and love were tangible. At the end of the meeting, I was allowed to ask one question of the group. I asked what the students' dreams were. One girl from Detroit had lost 90 pounds, and she wanted to become a physician in order to help other children. One boy had lost 100 pounds. He wanted to become a professional ballplayer. To my surprise, another student said, "Since you're 14 and you've never really played ball, you are not going to make it." The boy answered, "That doesn't matter; it's about what happens to me on the way that counts."

Of course, most kids who need help cannot access this type of program. "Think smaller," school principals told me.

THINKING SMALL(ER): THE CLASSROOM OF THE FUTURE

A smaller-scale solution fell into my lap in 2008. One afternoon Shelly came into my office and told me that she was on the parent-teacher board of the elementary school her son attended. Shelly had worked in the lab for a decade and wanted *her* kids to get a NEAT education.

Soon after that, by coincidence, I was invited to an organization called A Chance to Grow in Minneapolis; it was a rehabilitation center housed inside a school. Its leaders were intrigued by our School of the Future concept; they had, in essence, been doing a similar thing, but they had been more focused on integrating childhood physical rehabilitation with education.

A Chance to Grow was run by Bob DeBoer. He greeted us from his wheelchair with a giant smile. I followed him into the heart of the school, a large, high-ceilinged warehouse-like space with rubber flooring. It reminded me of our School of the Future. Throughout the space were 20-foot contraptions built largely from wooden 2" x 4" beams. Attached to the contraptions were springs and pulleys that held hammock-like devices. Each piece of equipment was designed to accentuate a certain type of movement. Climbing frames had an obvious function. The pulley-and-hammock system enabled children with specific disabilities to be supported while moving. Overall, it looked like an advanced Pilates gym. In this space, children completed physical therapy while being educated at the same time. For example, while clambering across a climbing frame, a child would be taught mathematics. While bouncing between demarcated circles with letters printed on them, kids completed spelling challenges. The Pilates-like space was completely integrated with learning. For most of the school day, children would learn in normal classrooms. For one or two periods, they would come to this exotic space.

I said to Bob, "Let's collaborate."

The School of the Future had intrigued many teachers around the country, but many also expressed frustration that they could not use this approach due to its cost. A Chance to Grow provided an alternate model. Rather than building an entire school, we could redesign one classroom in every school, a chair-free space where children could receive NEAT education. Inside the classroom, we could install an adapted version of the Pilates-like equipment and so promote NEAT movement. Rather than kids being in the classroom all the time, they could visit the NEAT classroom for one or two periods each day. Sure, this was not a total immersion, but it was better than nothing. On Shelly's urging, we decided to pilot the idea at her son's school.

Bamber Valley Elementary School is at the edge of Rochester, where the cornfields meet the city. The school is a one-story building with an open floor plan. The hallways are bright and decorated with student art. But what struck me the most about Bamber Valley was the transparent happiness of the students—this was a happy school. When we visited, Shelly and I were instructed to wait outside the principal's office on tiny orange plastic chairs.

I grew up in London, and Mrs. Brewster ran my elementary school in military style. All interactions with Mrs. Brewster were terrifying. As I sat outside Principal Gerdes's office on the tiny orange chair, those feelings came back. I began to sweat.

Soon we were ushered in. Everything I remembered about Mrs. Brewster was the opposite with Principal Gerdes. I felt I had entered the office of my favorite aunt. Principal Gerdes had a giant smile, and I half expected her to offer us freshly baked cookies. Instead, she offered her help. She immediately designated a large classroom that would become the Classroom of the Future. She also knew which teachers would be the most receptive to having their children use it. She explained that although she could make all of the logistics happen, we first would need to convince the parents.

The following Wednesday evening, Shelly and I returned to the school. In the school library, a table had been laid with drinks, chips and cookies. About a dozen parents showed up. Shelly and I began our presentation. The room felt tense until Principal Gerdes walked in. Her presence was enough; the parents, one after another, agreed to their children using the Classroom of the Future once a day. We held a second parent meeting a week later with a similar positive response.

Ms. Gerdes arranged for a large classroom to be emptied. We worked closely with A Chance to Grow, and, spending about $500, we built the Pilates-like wooden equipment complete with climbing frames, jumping mathematics boards and a variety of other learning equipment. The school inspector approved the safety features, and the Mayo Ethics Committee approved the approach. We met with the janitorial staff to make sure they were okay with this strange-looking Classroom of the Future. The most notable thing about it was that there were no chairs.

It was agreed that the students in Mrs. Waltz's class would be the test class; she was thrilled, but not as much as the kids—they loved the idea! All the kids started wearing our MEMS accelerometer activity sensors before the Classroom of the Future was opened. This baseline period lasted two weeks; during this time, the kids would use their normal classroom and normal chairs; they drove us crazy asking when they could start using the Classroom of the Future.

After two weeks, the fun began. The students used the Classroom of the Future for one 45-minute period per day. In the Classroom of the Future, the kids continued to wear the MEMS NEAT activity sensors, and Ms. Gerdes insisted that they complete exhaustive state-of-the-art educational tests.

The results exceeded all of my hopes. The MEMS sensors showed that student movement increased dramatically while they used the Classroom of the Future for the 45-minute period, as expected. But the impact of the 45-minute class extended far beyond that one period. Students were more active for the rest of the day. We compared recess time before and after the experiment began: when kids used the Classroom of the Future, they sat less and moved more during recess too. Not only did their NEAT activity increase for the day they used the Classroom of the Future, but it carried forward into the following morning. In fact, using a NEAT classroom for only 45 minutes per day increased a student's activity for more than 36 hours. It was as if we had kindled a fire inside of these kids. The increased NEAT levels were not as great as with the $500,000 School of the Future program in which students were immersed all day, but what a return for $500! The good news didn't stop there. State educational scores improved, as did the detailed educational assessments in mathematics and spelling.

It seemed that we didn't need to rebuild every school in America, but rather build *Classrooms* of the Future in every school and ensure that students can access them as part of their curriculum. If kids move their bodies, their minds move too.

But we weren't quite done.

THINKING TINY: JUST GIVE ME FIVE MINUTES

A colleague asked me if I could think of a project for her daughter Vanessa, who was completing her master's in education. I went to see Shelly. We had just completed analyzing all of the Bamber Valley data, and I assumed that Shelly was battle weary—working with kids is rewarding but exhausting. But when I asked Shelly if she wanted to do more, she almost jumped out of her chair and exclaimed, "Yes!" Soon afterward Vanessa came to the lab.

Shelly explained to Vanessa that although the studies at Bamber Valley were conducted on seven- to eight-year-olds, she suspected that we needed to prevent chair addiction at a younger age. She explained that the motor strip in the brain that drives limb movements becomes set at around the age of five. Prior to that age, the brain is at its most fluid, so the earlier we intervene to prevent chair-habituation, the better.

We had learned from Bamber Valley that you don't necessarily need to completely redesign the entire building but rather the implicit *structure* of education—like changing corporate culture. If movement can be built into education as part of the curriculum, not only will students learn better, they also will be healthier. The Bamber Valley study suggested that seven- to eight-year-olds only needed to add 45 minutes of active learning into their school day to benefit. Shelly wondered whether the intervention could be even shorter in younger children.

Vanessa joined the lab brimming with enthusiasm. She was already working with preschoolers as part of her thesis, and she came up with an idea that was so simple I was certain it would fail. She wrote down a series of five-minute activities on small pieces of paper. The activities included jumping up and down while reciting letters, running around a geography map and singing while bouncing. She put the pieces of paper in an empty jar and took it to the preschool. At times throughout the day, the teacher would pull one activity out of the jar and have the kids act it out. With the agreement of the parents, the children wore our MEMS activity sensors.

The sensors confirmed that NEAT increased during the five-minute active breaks, so we knew that the preschoolers were compliant. But like the Bamber Valley experiment, the effect of these five-minute active breaks impacted the rest of the day; overall, the kids moved 30 percent more! Again we collected detailed educational data, and the children in the five-minute NEAT program learned better, especially their letters.

ACTIVE LEARNING: ALL POSITIVES

Other labs conducted multiple studies to confirm the benefits of active learning. News circled back to the White House, and First Lady Michelle Obama launched her "Let's Move" campaign (http://www.letsmove.gov). The results were so consistent that a National Forum on Active Learning was founded in 2013. Over the last decade, much has been learned about NEAT-active education:

1. If you give students the opportunity to move throughout the day, they will do so.
2. When students move more, their education improves.
3. The more you move, the better you learn.
4. Children are happier and experience less stress in NEAT-activated education.
5. Classroom behavior improves with active learning.
6. Children who move more have greater creativity.

When you think about it, these findings make perfect sense. The connection between learning and moving is encoded in our DNA.

But the gloves have got to come off. Today a third of US youth are overweight or have obesity; that's 23 million kids.[10] Since 1980, obesity rates among children have tripled. In health centers across America, pediatricians are seeing increased rates of asthma and joint problems. Children are now developing adult diseases while in school: diabetes, fatty liver disease, hypertension and even cardiovascular disease. Not for a second am I claiming that the chair sentence is the entire cause of childhood obesity or that school is the only culprit. However, what is clear is that the chair sentence is even more lethal in children than adults; a teenager with obesity has an 80 percent chance of carrying the excess weight into adulthood. Validated and sustainable school solutions exist for reversing lethal sitting in children. Insist on change.

13

GET UP!, STEP 1

Get Personal!

HAVING A CHAIRLESS OFFICE, HOME OR SCHOOL HELPS only if you get up.

If I have not convinced you of the harmfulness of sitting, you must be in denial or seduced beyond sense by your chair. Getting off your bottom is a simple matter—you can do it right now! But changing sitting behavior long term is a greater challenge.

Over the next few chapters, I am going to share with you some of the secrets of how to escape lethal sitting and so win the war against The Chairman. These chapters are not meant to be a step-by-step manual, but I hope the concepts will help.

The first step is to appreciate that in the same way the chair sentence is a personal affliction, so too must be the solution. There are only three reasons a person does something: the cue, the response and the reward.

The cue is the stimulus to do something; you might not think you want a piece of candy until somebody offers you one. The response is something you've learned to do; when somebody offers you the candy, you reach out, take it and say thank you.

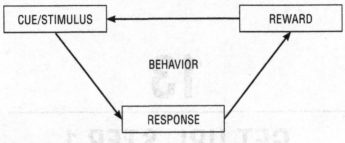

The triad of human behavior

The reward is the sweet taste in your mouth, the sugar high and also perhaps a memory from childhood when your dad gave you a candy.

With sitting, the cues are everywhere. We are drenched in sit cues: "Come and sit down." There are chairs everywhere. But the cues to sit are more profound than the simple availability of chairs. Human functioning has become chair-based; you cannot keep your job unless you sit in front of the computer screen all day. You cannot socialize on Sunday with your friends unless you join them on the sofa to watch football. You cannot have friends at school unless you play video games in the basement. Rather than cooking together, we get drive-through meals together.

Because the cues to sit are so ubiquitous, it is easy to understand that the response "I'll sit" is inescapable.

The reward system for sitting all day long is equally overt. Broadly speaking, rewards that excite people feed into one of their three primal drives: money, sex and power. And so the hedonist's behavioral cycle is set—sitting begets pleasure, so we sit more.

Ultimately every behavior you participate in is your own. Of course, constraints are placed on us much of the time, but how you *respond*—your behaviors—is up to you.

MAKE SENSE

By now you should recognize that the chair-based lifestyle we have gravitated to has hurt not just our bodies but our minds and spirits as well. Getting up from a life of sedentariness is akin to leaving a mind-numbing prison.

The chair-based existence is essentially one of sensory deprivation. Seated all day and all evening, we deprive ourselves of organic smells, three-dimensional sights, live sound, home-cooked tastes and human touch. Experiments performed in light-deprived cats demonstrated that the structure and function of cats' brains contracted with sensory deprivation (chapter 3). This must also be true in humans who spend a lifetime sitting. And so, as we begin to walk again, it is necessary to (1) control the stimuli we expose ourselves to, (2) alter our responses to chair-based cues and (3) ensure that rewards we strive for are valuable enough to us.

CHAIRS ARE MASS PRODUCED
BUT PEOPLE ARE NOT

If I could describe myself as having four traits, I would relate one to each of my four grandparents: scientist (Grandpa Poppa), nurturer (Grandma Jesse), educator (Grandpa Danny) and artist (Grandma Gags). I did not select these four elements; rather, they are part of my DNA. Our personalities are imprinted by about the age of two. Just like our physical features, they define who we are.

LESSONS FOR THE SOVIET MILITARY

Ivan Petrovich Pavlov, working in the 1890s at the Institute of Experimental Medicine in St. Petersburg, was the Soviet Union's father of modern psychology. He was also Professor of Pharmacology at the Military Medical Academy where the Soviet military machine was investing heavily in understanding the psychology of soldiers. According to the Academy's research, each person had one of 16 distinct personality types imprinted from birth.[1] The Soviets viewed understanding a soldier's personality type as critical to how a person was effectively deployed in a military organization. To illustrate the importance of these personalotypes, as I call them, let's examine two: Heroic Risk Taker and Calm Organizer.

If the military objective is to take a bridge during a battle, you need to deploy a Heroic Risk Taker—someone who is courageous and prepared to go in alone and lead from the front; in this situation, the Calm Organizer would be useless.

In warfare, there needs to be a person in charge of supplies and ammunitions. This person is critical because a war will be lost if the soldiers are unfed and without bullets. You want the Calm Organizer to be in charge of supplies and ammunitions; the Heroic Risk Taker would be useless.

Personalotypes, much like the traits I inherited from my grandparents, are to a degree woven into our DNA.[2] These traits follow us throughout our lives. Your personalotype may have broader implications than simply affecting your behavior; for instance, it can impact your health. Consider obesity, which has a significant genetic component[3]; the DNA of your personality may be the critical genetic element. Imagine that a woman's DNA makes her a Heroic Risk Taker and that she is given a desk job in an insurance firm. Being confined to repetitive tasks—and to a chair—is contrary to the DNA of a Heroic Risk Taker. Imagine the angst she feels working in the insurance company. Not only is she not very good at her job, always arguing and somewhat disorganized, but when she gets home, her anxiety results in comfort eating and the need to escape reality through alcohol.

On the face of it, you might think that a chair sentence is perfect for the Calm Organizer personalotype. Think back to the Soviet army. Imagine the Calm Organizer carrying crates of bullets and storing them in a carefully designated part of a beautifully organized storage warehouse. Next the Calm Organizer brings in boxes of canned meat. He stacks them elsewhere and carefully records the number of boxes. In the modern office, the Calm Organizer is burning 1,500 fewer calories/day than when organizing manually; his physicality also gets pent up. Even the

Calm Organizer was not designed to sit all day and slide a computer mouse around.

LETHAL SITTING—BAD FOR BODY, BAD FOR MIND

Imagine now, the Calm Organizer carrying a box of bullets into the warehouse. Someone calls to him, "Would you look at the map and choose a good bar for us to go to tonight?" "I'm busy. I'll do it later," he says.

Now imagine the same scenario in the modern insurance office. The Calm Organizer stops what he is doing, opens up Google, locates a nearby bar and emails the information to his coworker—*a purposeless distraction.*

Similarly, imagine our Heroic Risk Taker single-handedly capturing an enemy bridge. A friend calls out as she charges into the oncoming gunfire, "Could you choose an Italian restaurant for tonight?" The Heroic Risk Taker is hardly going to stop her assault. In the modern insurance office, the Heroic Risk Taker is already antsy—she is only too happy to embark on a *purposeless distraction.*

Distraction, wrote the philosopher Blaise Pascal in his book *Pensées,* is the source of all misery: "The reason that we distract ourselves from one thing . . . is that the present condition is inconsolably wretched." Modern research confirms that distraction degrades happiness; purposeless distraction makes people unhappy.[4]

The term "multitasking" was not originally coined to describe human activities. IBM engineers invented the word to describe the capacity of a modern computer to conduct multiple tasks simultaneously. Isn't it ironic that modern human beings are described as multitaskers? Try this: At the same time, rub your tummy and hammer a nail into a wall. The human is not designed to multitask.

Modern office workers are essentially forbidden to work all morning on a single project and ignore their emails. Many modern workers continuously function in a "drop this—do that" workflow—as soon they start something, they are told to stop it. Multitasking has spread far beyond the office, however. How often have you sat down for a meal and seen people answering their texts or cell phones? Multitasking, the *Harvard Business Review* has reported, is associated with a drop in IQ of 11 points.[5] This is the equivalent of working without a night's sleep or working while smoking marijuana. Productivity falls by about 40 percent in workers who multitask. Is it a surprise that frenetic task chopping diminishes the product?

WE EACH HAVE A DISTINCT personalotype that may explain an array of traits:

- Whether we are Heroic Risk Takers or Calm Organizers
- How we respond to certain situations (e.g., are you a comfort eater?)
- Whether we are disposed to smile or to frown
- How we process stimuli
- Whether we like to learn visually or through books

Just as people's tastes for music, art and food vary, your personalotype will affect how your chair escape unfolds. Some people like to play competitive sports; others enjoy yoga. Some people like to train for marathons; others like to mall walk. I know a 36-year-old woman who left her cubicle job and started her own company because she felt confined, both physically and intellectually. Today this Heroic Risk Taker is happier and 30 pounds lighter. I know a 45-year-old financial services executive who constructed his own intricate treadmill desk; this highly successful Calm Organizer is happier and 25 pounds lighter. Because we are unique and glorious human creations, respect your personalotype—one chair escape cannot fit all.

14

GET UP!, STEP 2

Plan!

THE BRITISH MUSEUM, IN THE HEART OF CENTRAL LONDON, is home to the world's oldest known chair. It is about 5,000 years old and is Egyptian. In stark contrast to the mass-produced modern office chair, the world's first chair, Chair Zero, was made from ebony and had ivory trim and an ivory seat. Scenes depicting wars and everyday events were carved into the ivory. Interestingly, these carvings show only standing Egyptians walking, manually farming with tools and fighting on their feet; the default body posture was standing. The chair was respite from a day spent otherwise up and moving.

WAGING CHAIR WAR

If the chair has truly become an enemy, in order to get up, we need a strategic plan to defeat it. Sun Tzu was a Chinese general in the Zhou Dynasty about 2,500 years ago. A book attributed to him is on the bookshelf of many corporate managers and sports coaches: *The Art of War*. Sun Tzu's first principle of war is to develop a detailed assessment and plan.

Winning the chair war is a matter of life or death. Therefore, you cannot undertake this war without careful and deep reflection. I will repeat: The chair war is a matter of life or death. Intricate planning is necessary.

WAR PLAN

The chair war requires you to plan for five fundamental factors that are essential for a victorious campaign.

Part 1: Terrain

To win your war, what terrain do you need to travel to ultimately overcome your chair sentence? Let's start with you—your *personal* terrain. What psychological hang-ups do you need to overcome? Are you afraid that if you pace around the office, people will think you are strange? Are you afraid that if you ask your partner to go for a walk this evening, you might actually connect and have a good time? Do you feel self-conscious about your weight? Go on. Dig inside. What *personal* terrains must you overcome? Are they parents, your marriage, coworkers or the person who stares back at you from the mirror? What five things about yourself would you most like to change?

1. _____
2. _____
3. _____
4. _____
5. _____

This list is your *personal* terrain. The critical barrier—the one you must address *now*—is the first item on this list.

Next you need to assess your *physical* terrain: home, work and leisure areas. What barriers must you get around? Some barriers are imaginary. For example, you do not need a treadmill to get off your bottom while watching TV; your boss may be happy to have walk-and-talk meetings with you *if you ask*. (You may want to sweeten the deal; walk-and-talk meetings are 11 minutes shorter on average.)

Part 2: Seasons

Animals are seasonal. Squirrels hide nuts in fall; huskies grow thick coats in winter; bears hibernate. The pineal gland is the part of the brain that modulates how mammals respond to the seasons. The human is seasonal too, but in the modern flurry of heated/air-conditioned living, we've forgotten the natural pace of nature.

One afternoon in 2010, Gabe asked me to come meet a student of his. "She's fantastic," he said. Samantha Calvin, in her 20s, from Raymond, Minnesota, was waiting for us in the conference room. She was in a business suit, pacing nervously. Most students show up in jeans and T-shirts.

Samantha, in her first year in college, gave a presentation a PhD would be proud of. She wanted to understand why refugees from Somalia were developing obesity and diabetes. In Somalia, she explained, people were farmers and lived seasonally, being active in peak agricultural times and resting off-season. In these agricultural communities, food production just meets energy needs and people stayed thin. Samantha hypothesized that when the Somalian farmers stopped farming and came to the United States, they gave up 2,500 NEAT calories per day and ate low-cost, high-fat processed foods—the perfect storm for obesity. Samantha proved to be right. She has been with the lab ever since.

A year later Samantha called another meeting for the lab to attend. This presentation was even more polished than the first; she explained that rates of obesity, diabetes and cardiovascular disease are far higher in American Indian/Alaska Native populations (39 percent obesity rate) than non-Hispanic whites (24 percent).[1] She suggested that there were parallels to what she had been investigating with the Somalian refugees. Samantha suggested that American Indian populations were used to living seasonally and that modernity had completely disrupted this pattern of living. And so, she wanted to work in partnership with an American Indian reservation to prevent obesity by reversing harmful sitting and promoting NEAT. A month later Samantha began working with the Mille Lacs Reservation in central Minnesota.

The Mille Lacs Reservation (*Misi-zaaga'iganiing* in the Ojibwe language) covers 61,000 acres and includes three communities: Mille Lacs, East Lake and Lake Lena. The seasons here transition from a long arctic winter through gentle spring and hot humid summer to colorful fall. The people who live at Mille Lacs now watch the seasons from their modern homes spread across the reservation. It was not always this way.

Tribal ancestors used to move homes based on the seasons. Winter homes were covered with skins and kept warm by a central fire. Spring homes were located by the water for planting wild rice and fishing. Summer homes were located in tree shade and were accessible to game-rich land. Fall homes facilitated food storage and tanning of skins. Activities requiring high NEAT levels occurred in the warm months, when food was plentiful. When less food was available in winter, people were more sedentary.

Frances Mabel Staples, who is a Mille Lacs Band elder, talked about her childhood:

> I was born on June 30, 1928 at a summer campsite in the woods.
> They did logging there and picked rutabagas when it was ruta-
> baga season . . . We had to work all the time, help our parents
> outside in the heat and sun. We used to wash socks on one of
> those washboards. That was tough duty . . . We hauled wood, cut
> it up. . . . We shook that rice and it came out clean.[2]

Frances's existence was tethered to nature and packed with arduous daily NEAT activities. Frances moved throughout her day as nature demanded and rested when the work and season allowed. In the world Frances describes, the default body posture is up and moving. Now, 80 years later, the default is to sit.

As our links to nature loosen, our bodies lose that natural pacing. Nature dictates that there are times to sit—mostly when the weather inhibits activity and the food supply is low. The rest of the year, though, nature demands that we are active so that we don't starve.

In other populations that live in tune with nature, sitting also follows seasonality. Among Gambian farmers, for instance, peak agricultural activity increases calorie burn two and a half times above the number of calories expended in the rest period of the year.[3]

Can this natural association with nature be found in the developed world? I went to visit a nature school in Sweden, where student education is directly linked to the seasons. Biology lessons are conducted outside; students write poetry and learn English in the woods and do mathematics while jumping between stones across the river. The children are high achieving, in tune with nature and healthy.

Humans are not designed to ignore the natural pace of the world we live in.

But there is more to seasons than weather—it is in the nature of all things to exhibit periods of high- and low-intensity activity. One of the greatest mistakes people make when trying to advance in life, whether their business, career, education, wealth or health, is failing to understand that it is natural that efforts should pulse over time. The only time that urgency occurs in nature is when there is imminent danger to life or body; in nature there is no such thing as an emergency email. Plan for the natural rhythm of change: a PhD can take five years to complete; credit card debt, two years to pay off; and a good marriage grows like a tree over decades. You will not go from chair sentenced to free in one moment. As your body readjusts to moving the way it was designed to move, the ropes that bind you to your chairs will slowly melt away.

Part 3: Leadership

Another mistake often made by people trying to change their lives is to feel that they have to *lead* the campaign. This is not necessary. For example, a tech executive who is a successful leader in her business may not be the best leader for her evening kick-boxing class. In planning your chair escape, you may need to lean on the leadership of others. I am awful at filling out forms and so rely on the leadership of my accountant to file my taxes correctly. When I see patients with obesity who have had an abuse history, who have depression or who are in dire financial straits, I advise them to seek professional help (i.e., the leadership of others) before starting a weight management program. If you relate to this, please seek the leadership of a professional right away. (For immediate help, call the 24/7 National Suicide Prevention Lifeline at 1-800-273-8255. Your local library has resources for getting help with financial restructuring). To be free of your chair sentence, let someone else lead you. At the end of the day, you will be victorious.

Part 4: Time and Resource Management

How will your chair war be organized? Time management and resource management are critical. A client told me, "I have a gym at work but never use it." This is an example of both poor time management and poor resource management.

Do you remember the Filofax revolution in the 1980s? Filofaxes were A4-sized, hyperfashionable paper-based personal organizers and day-planners. Yuppies would not be seen in public without their Filofaxes! It became chic to have your calendar, contacts, notes, priorities and lists meticulously organized and color-coded. Being organized was in! Organized people get stuff done. A critical part of your great chair escape is to get organized.

A client in Boston told me that she wanted to try yoga but could not afford it. Within ten minutes I found five places in Boston where she could try a yoga class for free; I found a series of six community education classes for $14, and the local Y charged $30 a month for membership and offered yoga four times a week. She agreed to convert her daily Venti Caramel Latte to a Short Cappuccino. She paid for her Y membership simply by reorganizing her coffee preference; her stress, calorie intake and dress size fell. This is an example of an effective allocation of resources, but it required (ten minutes) planning.

In another example, a woman in her 40s came to talk with me at a free clinic in Mesa, Arizona. She wanted to be more active but could not afford a gym. I asked her what type of activity she liked most. She immediately replied, "Years ago, I used to have a dog called Zelda, but she died. I'd love to have a dog, but I can't afford it." Within five minutes the two of us had contacted the Arizona Animal Welfare League, a no-kill dog shelter. They had a volunteer dog-walking program; she agreed to begin training the following day. This was a simple, no-cost solution, but it took (five minutes) thought and planning.

Planning does not need to take hours, but to win a war, you must have a plan, and the better your plan, the more chance you have to win.

Part 5: The Map

Warfare is dynamic. A battle can change in an hour. You have to nimbly respond to offensive forces. Winning a war is not a matter of following a straight line step by step or day by day; you must be adaptable. Imagine that you are going to a basketball game tonight. You get on the highway, and it is jammed because of a car wreck. You can either inflexibly sit in the jam and miss the game or find an alternate route. Adaptability is a key part of your strategy for escaping the chair.

Consider that you're trying to get from where you are now (Point A) to a place five miles away (Point B). If you look on a map, you'll see that there are numerous ways to get there. Similarly, if your chair is Point A and your new active life is Point B, there are numerous routes you can take to reach your goal. Set off on one route, but if you meet a roadblock, you can either be rigid and fail, or adapt and win.

The objective of your chair escape plan is to reach Point B, the new dynamic. Yes, carefully plan your chair escape but understand that to win the war, you will need to adapt as you go. Never fear; there are multiple ways to reach your destination, some of which you have not yet even considered.

Time and time again, whether it is in business or in warfare, commanders fail to win by not having a plan. To overthrow The Chairman you will need a strategic plan. Anticipate:

1. The terrain you have to navigate
2. The seasonality—the ups and downs—of the human spirit
3. The necessity to find leaders and guides to help you
4. Be efficient with your time and resources. Invest five minutes of planning time per day on your chair escape
5. There are many ways to reach your destination: be adaptable

You can overcome lethal sitting. You can overcome the modern sedentariness of spirit, mind and body. You can defeat the The Chairman. Plan on it!

15

GET UP!, STEP 3

Weapons!

HERE ARE THE FIVE WEAPONS YOU NEED TO ESCAPE CHAIR
bondage.

WEAPON 1: CUE AND STIMULUS CONTROL

If I don't go to the mall, I won't spend money. If I don't buy cookies and have them in the house, I'm less likely to eat them. With
respect to reversing the chair sentence, if I don't prioritize a salsa
dance lesson at 4 p.m., I'm less likely to attend it. If I get home
on Friday without *any* weekend plans, I am unlikely to get off my
recliner. If I put the treadmill in the TV room, I am more likely
to walk while watching TV. If I leave rubber bands on my desk, I
am more likely to use them during the workday.

We are besieged by cues and stimuli to sit; controlling the
stream of sedentary stimuli is key.

WEAPON 2: SOCIAL SUPPORT

Social support—a person to lean on and move with—is a critical weapon. Human beings are social animals. The number one

question I asked my kids when they got back from school was "What did you learn?" The number one thing they told me was about their friends or foes. Social support is as critical to going for a walk at lunchtime as it is for having healthy foods at home. If my wife is trying to pay off our credit card bill and I go out and buy a big-screen TV, that is one failed support system!

WEAPON 3: SELF-MONITORING

If I am trying to pay off my car or credit card loan, I keep track of and monitor my bank account. The second tool to reverse the chair sentence is self-monitoring. A host of devices and apps can help; for instance there are devices that measure your activity level and apps that let your track your calorie expenditure and intake. It is important to recognize that if you are changing your sitting behavior, you must monitor your effectiveness.

WEAPON 4: REWARD SYSTEM

Think of the power of frequent flyer miles, coupon clipping, having platinum status and the never-ceasing series of reward programs. One of my clients who worked for an air-conditioning company could not get his head around quitting smoking. I got him into a quit program and told him to put all his cigarette money *in cash* into a vase. Almost 18 months later, I received a postcard from him. He was in Hawaii. He had paid for it with ash cash!

Remember from chapter 13 that the most successful reward systems feed into the primal drives: money, sex and power.

Reward systems are powerful. Earn it, love it!

WEAPON 5: COGNITIVE RESTRUCTURING

The fourth weapon you need is cognitive restructuring. Psycho-babble? No way! Cognitive restructuring is a powerful weapon that involves changing the inner voice—the voice that puts you down far too often—inside your head. "How can I ever get myself out of debt? I'm a spender!" If that is what a person thinks, you know he is doomed to fail. "How can I ever ask him out? He's out of my league!" Will she *ever* get up enough courage to ask him out? You know the answer! By changing that inner voice, you change your *response* to the cues and stimuli that drive behavior.

The trouble is, changing your inner voice, while theoretically simple, is really a big challenge.

Clients who are overweight tell me: "I feel so bad when I go out," "I feel ugly," "She does not want me." The reality is that this is *all* said by the internal voice inside your head. There are no facts to substantiate it!

I had a strange experience recently. I was supposed to have a professional meeting with a woman who had an idea for a program she wanted to start. Just before I hung up from talking with her, I said (I don't know why), "By the way, I'll be in a suit and tie"—my standard business attire. Just before the meeting, she texted me: "I did not tell you. I'm a large woman and don't feel like dressing up." She never came to the meeting.

Cognitive restructuring has three elements: positive self-speak, visualization and action response. To start cognitive re-structuring, spend one minute (use a timer) each morning in front of the mirror and say good things to your self; deliberately silence that negative inner voice. Before you leave your home, glance in the mirror; do you look as good as you can? If not, upgrade your appearance. You may think that this positive self-speak is a little "out there," but executives, actors and sports stars use this technique. One minute of positive self-speak is a strong way to start the day, but throughout the day you need to continue asserting your positive inner voice and pushing back the negative. The more you hear positivity inside, the stronger you become; you are strengthening your self-respect muscle.

Slalom skiers visualize the entire ski course in their minds before they leave the start gate; the technique is called visualiza-tion. Visualization is widely used in sports, and it is the next step in cognitive restructuring. Take the example that you want to ask your boss to change your weekly meeting into a walk-and-talk meeting. Imagine your boss standing in front of you, and rehearse the request several times in your head. You'll find that when you actually make the request, it will easily roll off your tongue. Visualization is useful for asking someone out on a date, requesting a raise or having a tough discussion with your spouse.

The third element in cognitive restructuring is to take the first step. This could be as simple as getting out of your chair at lunchtime to walk, getting the telephone number of the person you want to ask out or printing off the information for a course you want to take. After positive self-speak and visualization, your body has to feel an action response.

Cognitive restructuring is a central weapon you'll need for reversing all aspects of sedentariness. Through cognitive restructuring, you *can* silence that negative inner voice. Get up and move!

FIVE WEAPONS, ONE MISSION

The five weapons: cue and stimulus control, social support, self-monitoring, reward systems and cognitive restructuring are powerful enforcers of the cue-response-reward cycle that is the basis of human behavior.

CAUTIONARY TALES

The five weapons just described are powerful. As with any weapons, you have to be careful how you use them.

Cautionary Tale 1: Cue and Stimulus Control

We receive negative cues and stimuli from being around the wrong people. The expression "hanging out with the wrong crowd" exemplifies the importance of avoiding negative social

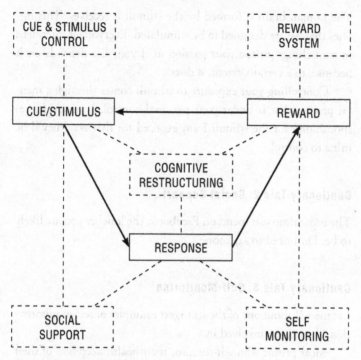

How the five weapons relate to behavior

stimuli. If your best friend sits in front of the TV or computer every night, you are more likely to sit when the two of you get together. The people we spend most of our time with—whether spouse, friend, coworker or relative—have the greatest power to alter the stimuli we are exposed to.

If you want to win your chair war, spousal support is critical.[1] If your spouse is your prison guard, get counseling.

The other cautionary note about stimulus control is to ensure that we get the stimuli we need. I have heard the same expression from a 17-year-old, an executive, a homemaker and a factory worker. The expression is "I'm so bored." To alleviate that boredom, the 17-year-old smoked marijuana, the executive drank alcohol and the homemaker and factory worker used narcotics.

The human brain is formed by the stimuli it receives. This implies that we are designed to be stimulated. Everyone is interested in something; pursue your passion as if your life depends on it because, to a certain extent, it does.

Controlling your exposure to stimuli comes through a mental process that is under your personal control. I must take responsibility for the stimuli I am exposed to; that way they'll be mine to control.

Cautionary Tale 2: Social Support

The more time you spend on Facebook, the lonelier you are likely to be. Do I need to say more?

Cautionary Tale 3: Self-Monitoring

Let me tell about one of the strangest examples of self-monitoring that I have been involved in.

Most people who self-monitor their health keep lists of their blood test results, the foods that they eat or the number of steps they take. When I was a medical student, I was involved in a more unusual monitoring system.

WARNING: *If you are about to eat something, put it back in the fridge.*

One summer, a friend of mine, Richard Fox, was desperate to find another medical student who could fill in as a mentor at a summer high school science program.

I volunteered because the program provided free room and board in the English countryside for two months. Each mentor was assigned a group of enthusiastic science-oriented students. Our job was to devise a scientific project with them, gather data and present it at a high school conference at the end of summer.

After much discussion with my group, we agreed to do something in nutrition. One of the consistent failures of the modern Western diet is a lack of fiber. Paucity of dietary fiber has been associated with impaired immunity and colon cancer. We decided to examine how stool might change with different doses of fiber supplementation.

Thereafter, the students started to take increasing doses of fiber supplements and to monitor the changes.

I learned a great deal about self-monitoring over these eight weeks. Several students didn't bother to measure their stool at all—this was because the measurement system (a paper tape measure dropped into the toilet bowl) was too irksome for them to use. Other students, at first, seemed to ardently measure their stool length but over time became sloppy; some of these students fessed up to falsifying their poop data. However, a third group of students were highly motivated for the entire project. They monitored their stool length with almost religious zeal and provided additional information regarding color and consistency. I remember one girl in particular who became angry to the point of screaming at her peers when they did not follow the protocol.

These three groups of students represent the limitations of self-monitoring. The first issue is that the measurement system has to be easy to apply and use. In the laboratory, we constantly find that writing things down, whether it concerns food intake, sitting time or feelings, is fraught with inaccuracy and recorder fatigue. Even those who feel invested in the process and record avidly at the beginning trail off after just a few weeks.

Self-monitoring fatigue is particularly relevant in regard to pedometer use. I have deployed pedometers in numerous corporate programs where we rely on individuals to write down their step counts and/or put the data into a computer system. Here is what happens: You get good data for the first few weeks, but then self-reporting drops off exponentially. You might think that this is simply the effect of having to write things down or remember to enter the data, but this is not so. Even when the device keeps the data itself and simply has to be swiped against the computer system, the mass self-gathering of data is usually short term.

Two reasons account for this finding. The first is that unless data have some value to users, they are worthless and so people stop gathering them. The second reason people stop self-monitoring after a few weeks is that they have learned what they need to do to reach their goal.

In our corporate studies, we use NEAT (nonexercise activity thermogenesis) MEMS accelerometer measurement devices that are lightweight and accurate and have simple data-download interfaces and attractive data displays. Despite making it as easy as possible to use the MEMS devices and record the data, what we found was that people self-monitor their sit time for about three weeks religiously. By then, most people recognize what they need to do to maintain low sit times and high activity times; thereafter, they stop using the device. What we've come to realize is that self-monitoring needs to span a distinct period of time to prevent user fatigue.

What I now suggest is that people follow a self-training period, using an activity tracker, for three weeks and then deliberately stop using it. During that three-week period they will work out what they need to do to decrease sitting time by, say, 20 percent. I then recommend that they continue their program and reuse the activity tracker three months later—like a car tune-up.

The other time to use their tracking device is when they take on a new challenge. For instance, say a client has an established pattern of walking ten minutes every hour while at work, and she now adds a one-hour walk in the evening. I recommend that she self-monitor with an activity device for the first three weeks of this new initiative so she can see data to affirm her success. Once this new pattern is established for 21 days, I tell her to put the tracker back in the drawer for another three months. Sun Tzu's thirteenth principle of war is to battle with intelligence. This is intelligent self-monitoring.

In our programs, we have run into self-monitoring addicts who love to measure themselves all the time. They will ignore this advice, but for the rest of us, this is a good approach to avoiding self-monitoring fatigue.

Cautionary Tale 4: Reward System

There is tremendous debate regarding how reward systems actually impact behavioral change. The most extreme example of a reward system that backfired was in a corporation I was consulting with in Delhi. The idea was to reward people for losing weight. The program was announced, and an excited buzz followed. However, during the time between the announcement and the start of the program, participants began to overeat like crazy. They wanted to begin the program at the maximum possible weight so that they could document greater weight loss and earn more money. Six months later, the program finished and winners received up to $100. Six months after that, the participants were weighed again: Many actually were heavier than when they started. In this example, the reward system actually did the participants harm.

A popular philosopher from Harvard asked a simple question: Is it right to bribe people to lose weight? He cited the example of a friend of his. Every time the friend's children wrote a thank-you note, he paid them $1. The philosopher noted that every time he visited his friend thereafter, he would receive several thank-you letters from the children. Although the thank-you letters were a good behavior, what is unknown was whether they conveyed true appreciation or whether the note writing would be sustained into adulthood. A bigger question concerns the philosophical implications of bribing children to behave politely. Most parenting organizations do not support the idea of paying your children to perform basic family tasks, such as carrying out the trash. It is interesting, however, that it is common in corporate health programs to reward people for doing what they should be doing anyway.

The most effective reward systems are self-driven. This is true for punishments too. I recently met a woman named Jessica, who told me that she connected her walk schedule to a Dickensian punishment system—if she did not complete her walk program every day for a month, she would not go on vacation. When I said to her that I thought that was extreme, she shrugged and said, "You have to commit." And, yes, she walked every day and went on vacation. This reward/punishment system suited *her*.

The more personalized and immediate your reward system is, the more it will help you escape your chair sentence. Reward systems that you implement are more powerful than systems overseen by others. The closer you can link *your* reward to *your* Get Up motion, the more reinforced that behavior becomes—at a neurological level. This is the reason that cocaine is so addictive; the high immediately follows the exposure. This is the most positively reinforcing reward system. Cocaine aside, learn from this cautionary tale. Build your own reward system so that you get a good buzz when you get up from your chair and a bigger sustained buzz once you *stay* out of it.

Cautionary Tale 5: Cognitive Restructuring

Julian is a remarkable man. He restructured the voice in his head and found himself kneeling in front of an open oven—ready to submit to the dark inside and kill himself.

Born a girl, Julian told me, "The moment I had an opinion of myself . . . always . . . I knew I was a boy." From the first moment he can remember, Julian felt he was a male in a female body. He described his childhood—physically as a girl—as "really happy." "I had everything, a great family and friends. I played sports, I was an athlete, I went to parties. I did everything presenting myself as a girl." Julian began to body build. He liked what the weights did to his body and became highly successful as a high school athlete. However, he explained that his brain was in "a fog." He knew he was meant to be a man—something was profoundly wrong with the status quo.

Inside, Julian knew there was anger. "Even as a young kid, in a minor way," but when puberty occurred, he said, "it exploded." At 16 years old, his anger—this internal conflict—"came out in torrents." He went through his first cognitive restructuring; the foggy person became an angry one.

At 18 he was given methamphetamine at a party. In an instant it numbed the pain; next, alcohol softened the edges. In his second cognitive restructuring, his internal voice yelled, "Do drugs. Take alcohol." About to be evicted from a cockroach-infested dump, he knelt before the oven and prayed to die.

When he hit bottom, Julian said "a spiritual awakening happened; it was profound," and he started to become what he truly wanted—a man. In that final cognitive reconstruction, the internal voice spoke truth. "There was change in my thinking that changed my life," he concluded. Julian is now successful in his career in medicine; he is also a public speaker and transgender advocate. In 2013 Julian was awarded *Echo* magazine's Man of the Year award.[2]

We learn from Julian that cognitive restructuring—for good—has to be done as a series of small self-nudges: "I will get up, switch off the TV/computer and take a short stroll tonight"; "I will try dating"; or "I will dress up and look good." Cognitive restructuring is a tool in your toolbox you can never leave behind. Speak to yourself with loving-kindness *all* the time.

LOOK, YOU ARE AT WAR. You need to carry your five weapons all the time. Never leave home without them:

Weapon 1. Cue and Stimulus Control
Weapon 2. Self-Monitoring
Weapon 3. Cognitive Restructuring
Weapon 4. Social Support
Weapon 5. Reward System

Be a great warrior; plan your campaign, gather your weapons, fight intelligently and win.

16

GET UP!, STEP 4

Play! The Pulse of Creativity

"YOU CAN DISCOVER MORE ABOUT A PERSON IN AN HOUR OF play than in a year of conversation," said Plato. What ever happened to kids playing in the playground, a stolen game of basketball at lunch and lovers strolling hand in hand? Play in childhood is necessary not only for physical development, but also for social and intellectual development. Adults play too. Play is a stress valve and a mechanism for socialization. I see people in our chair-release programs get up from their chairs and breathe fresh air into their lives. Play is a part of that. Sometimes you have to put aside your plan, weapons and standard operating procedures, let down your hair and play! Many of life's tragedies come unexpectedly. In the same way, so too should many of life's joys. Don't wait for a storm to pass; dash outside and dance in the rain. Don't let the chance to spontaneously tell someone you love them slip away; just say it! Get up, shake off the cobwebs and have some fun.

POVERTY PLAYGROUND

I was working in the Kibera slum in Nairobi trying to understand the interaction between people's NEAT (nonexercise activity thermogenesis) movement and poverty. Kibera is the world's second-largest slum. Working with local teams, we were planning the Kibera Mapping Project, where we would use advanced camera motion detection technologies to map both the slum spaces and alleyways (which are constantly changing) and also the movement of the 60,000 slum dwellers.

With my driver, JJ, I visited makeshift churches, spoke with people, hung out at beer stands and even got a haircut (tourist price!) at a barbershop with painted cardboard walls. It was filthy, hot and stank of sewage that flowed in open trenches.

One afternoon JJ and I sat in front of a beer hut next to a clearing and drank Tusker beer (tourist price). JJ was about my age, had two kids and an enormous smile. He understood that I did not like to talk and so was happy to drive me around for hours, walk through the alleyways, and hang out with me without saying a word. That afternoon we sat and drank beer. As we watched, a soccer match started on a nearby clearing.

There were about two dozen children playing. The goalposts were T-shirts and tree branches. The ball was a rusted tin can. The children played barefoot. We watched for more than an hour; JJ lay back on the wood platform that fronted the beer hut and fell asleep with a grin on his face.

The kids played. They ran, pushed, shoved, bossed each other around, cried and laughed. They celebrated goals and kicked at the yellow/red dust at missed opportunities. They laughed more than they cried. As the sun began to fall, the game stopped only because a riot broke out nearby over a stolen television, and JJ hustled me out of there.

I conducted similar studies in slums in Mumbai, India. One afternoon I was in a large slum close to the airport. Kids were at play there too. One of their favorite games was to jump on the back of commercial trucks, ride on them for a while and jump off. In another place a water main had broken, and two boys and a girl jumped, yelping and screaming with joy. Their happiness in the gushing water was identical to what I later saw at the water park in Wisconsin Dells—children soaked in fun.

Play is the domain of neither the rich nor the poor. It is the natural territory of childhood.

THE PLAY INSTITUTE

I met Dr. Stuart Brown, the director of the National Institute for Play, at a conference in Los Angeles. Stuart was balding, suntanned and happy. His lecture began with a series of photographs of playing children. Play, he argued, is essential for childhood development of the body and mind. I leaned back.

Stuart explained his link to the University of California, Los Angeles and an entire cadre of scientists. He did not show one or two studies but summary tables of scores of studies about the physical, psychological and social benefits of play.[1] He explained how play provided the bumps and stresses for healthy bone development, and he presented data on how play benefits cardiovascular fitness.[2]

Stuart went on to explain that, through play, children have been shown to develop physical coordination and improved math and spelling scores. He described how, with play, problem-solving thinking and IQ improve. He argued that the essence of creativity is born through play; that play itself is a creative process—just think of the innovated goalposts and tin-can football in Kibera and the jump-truck game in Mumbai.

But then the doctor went on to speak about socialization— how children learn to lead, and be led, through play. He spoke about how social structures are developed on the playground. When someone trips and falls, there is a natural caregiver. When someone kicks the ball over the fence, there is always one kid (the explorer) who goes to fetch it. There are loners, and there are mixers. There are cliques (the preemptor of political parties) and those who reject and are rejected by the cliques. There are winners and losers. The entire social structure is formed on the playground: love, hate, war, peace, leaders and the led.

PLAYGROUND GONE

Active three-dimensional play is vanishing from childhood. The chair has taken over. There are several reasons for this. First, and most obviously, there is the computer screen and video games. In 2012, more than one billion individuals played computer and video games.[3]

Video gaming emerged in the 1970s originally as an emulator of physical gaming; *Pong*, released in 1972, was an electronic table-tennis game, for instance. Electronic gaming improved along with home computers, and now, according to DFC Intelligence,[4] video gaming is a $66 billion per year industry that is expected to grow another 20 percent in the next four years. In China alone, online computer gaming is valued at $12 billion per year. Just as word processing has replaced handwriting, so has computer/video gaming displaced active outdoor gaming.

Electronic gaming has gained technical sophistication but lost social integrity. Computer games virtually arm children with weapons and help them visualize scenes of violence and sex they might have never encountered otherwise. In a school focus group in Iowa, a ten-year-old boy told me: "When I get stressed out, I go into the basement and shoot a whole bunch of people." He paused. "Then I feel a lot better."

As electronic gaming evolved, so too has addiction to it. Internet Gaming Disorder is now listed in the fifth edition of the *Diagnostic and Statistical Manual of Mental Disorders*.[5]

Massively multiplayer online role-playing games (MMORPG) is the technical term used to describe the most popular type of role-play web-based computer games, where large number of players role play with one another within a virtual world. This is how play is converted from physical interaction to an electronic interface. There are about 500 million MMORPG gamers strewn across the world; one game, *World of Warcraft,* has 8 million players worldwide.[6] Rates of addiction can be as high as 50 percent or as low as 1 percent of gamers, depending on the population being studied.[7] Chair-based, screen-based gaming no longer displaces only active outdoor play; it even displaces other sedentary activities, such as television watching. Children who play video games are more sedentary than even children who watch television.[8]

An extreme situation has emerged in Japan and South Korea, where some groups of children are so addicted to gaming that they do not leave their rooms or go to school. Instead, they have trained their parents to deliver food to their doors. Their rooms are dark and are fitted with wall-to-wall computer screens. These children have forgone all physical social connections; their world is artifice, and their bodies are crumbling as a consequence; 24 percent of these children require hospitalization to reverse their addiction.[9]

In Iowa City, I met an 11-year-old boy who plays *World of Warcraft* with peers across the world. The battles are scheduled at certain times, and, like a good soldier, he has to show up. The battles can start at 7 p.m., he told me, and end ten hours later. Once a B+ student, now he's failing. "I'm in the Army of the Dead. I've got hundreds of friends," he told me. "Any *living* friends?" I asked him. "Yeah," he replied, "they're all living." But gaming addiction is not limited to youth; Jeremy is a 38-year-old accountant who, because of his addiction to gaming, lost his marriage, children and job. He used gaming to escape from his real-life stressors.[10]

In addition to video and computer games, there are other reasons why play has mutated from active physical play to chair-based pursuits. We examined data for the Centers for Disease Control for sedentariness across more than 3,000 counties in the United States; these counties cover the majority of the nation's population.[11] People's zip codes predict how active they are. Those who live in a poverty-dense zip code—with higher rates of poverty and lower house prices—are four times more likely to be sedentary and to have obesity. Children living in poor areas sit more and engage less in active play. No one chooses to live in a poor neighborhood; perhaps personal choices have less to do with the chair sentence than we think.

BUT IT'S NOT JUST PLAY

Two victims of state school underfunding are physical education teachers and art teachers. I recently lectured at a high school in Minneapolis. There was no art teacher for a school of 800 students; instead, art had become IT. The kids had lessons using PowerPoint, Adobe and Microsoft Paint on computer screens. The tactile experience of molding clay or holding a brush was gone. Gone too was the mess of clay and the smell of paint. Gone were classroom clay fights when the teacher was not watching and the physical interaction of the body, hand and arm with art.

Think how a sculpture exists in three dimensions and how you can walk around it, touch it and smell it. It casts shadows as you move. I met an artist in her studio in Boston; she explained that she mixes infinite hues and shades of colors on her palette. As we spoke, I could smell the oil paint. Art on a flat computer screen, she told me, does not possess this dimension; colors are pixelated and selected from a predefined array of colors. You don't walk around a computer screen to admire computer art—you sit in front of it.

Human studies using functional magnetic resonance imaging scanners show that the brain formulates images differently from a computer screen compared to the free-living real world.[12] In the same way that video and computer play has become a flat experience, so too in art; sculptures and paintings created with pixels and PowerPoint are static, seated versions of what was once dynamic.

POVERTY CHAIR SENTENCE

I was intrigued with why poverty is such a driver of inactivity in US children (and adults); surely rich kids have greater access to video gaming, I thought. In 2011, I conducted focus groups in the Euclid area of Cleveland, one of the poorest parts of the city. After a few hours of talking with the first focus group, it was clear why poor kids play less and sit more. A mother said, "I don't let my kids play outside. They get involved in drugs or get shot." Before the evening was over, I heard five gunshot volleys.

At the time, there were streets in Cleveland where one out of three homes was going through foreclosure. Many deserted homes were falling into abject disrepair. Corporate collaborators had an idea to buy some of these homes (some were on sale for $20,000), level them and create local, neighborhood-based playgrounds. Houses were leveled, and supplies for playgrounds were brought in. In a few cases, all of the supplies were stolen from the vacant lots. Nonetheless, several playgrounds were built on these inner-city lots. I went to see one of them; it was empty. One mother told me that she would not let her kids play there even though it was only a five-minute walk from her house because the playground had become a center for drug dealing and was controlled by a local gang. "They [the drug dealers] love it," she said. "If the cops come, they run straight behind the houses at the back." In these neighborhoods, active play was too dangerous for kids to participate in. No wonder kids took to their chairs.

Paulette Baukol, from the Turtle Mountain Band of Chippewa Indians, set out to investigate whether it is lack of money or the inner-city urban jungle that has eroded childhood play.[13] She examined whether Native American kids living on open reservations are more active than Native American kids living in urban neighborhoods. Interestingly, she and her team discovered that children living on reservations are just as inactive as urban native kids. Native kids overall are less active than white children of similar age. I asked, "Why are children living on wide-open native reservations so inactive?" Paulette swung her long black hair and pierced me with a tight brown stare. "Do you know how dangerous some of our reservations are?" she asked. I looked blank. On some reservations, physical and sexual violence are unchecked, and drug and alcohol use are epidemic; these kids have nowhere safe to go.[14] The challenges in the urban environments are different to those on reservations; Native American kids living in urban areas cannot play in inner-city playgrounds because there is a hierarchy of violence. Native kids, who are at the bottom of the social order, get beaten up, mugged and shot the most often.[15] It is no wonder that parents do not let their kids play in the inner-city neighborhoods; for these children, television and game consoles are lifesavers.

If you want kids to play as they are meant to, you have to create safe places for them to do so. As I found out, the availability of land isn't the only requirement; the space must be safe and be kept safe. Critically, mothers in particular have to support efforts to keep their kids healthily active.

ACTIVE GAMING

Recognizing that millions of children are stuck in chairs playing only in virtual worlds, thought leaders began to ask in 2005 whether we could convert chair-based video gaming into active video gaming. If the answer was not throwing away the gaming console, maybe screen-based gaming could become active.[16]

I noticed that one scientific group in Hong Kong seemed ahead of many others. Chair-centric play is ubiquitous in Hong Kong, which is one of the most cramped and tech-rich cities in the world. Here not only is play space extremely limited, but video gaming carries social cachet. In Hong Kong, children's social status is determined more by their video game level than by the brand of shoes they wear.

I flew to Hong Kong to investigate. Dr. Alison McManus was the leader of the scientific group focused on active gaming. Judging by her resume, I expected a rather crusty academic. But no sooner had I arrived in Hong Kong on Sunday morning than Dr. McManus arranged a hike with her team up a local mountain trail; then she invited me to join her husband and kids for a swim at the beach.

That evening Alison invited me out for dinner. We sat, drank and ate. Suddenly someone rushed forward, and a camera flashed. "Dr. Levine, I caught you sitting," the man said. "I'm putting it up on Facebook." Even in Hong Kong, I could not escape The Chairman's reach!

Alison studied whether children could play video games while walking on a treadmill. The experiment generated fascinating insights. She discovered that children will *try* gaming while walking on a treadmill, but because they perceive that walking hurts their gaming skill, they often get off the treadmill and return to their seats.[17] The game comes first, and they'll subvert any system that threatens that. A better answer was needed.

Later that year, back in the United States, I was invited to be a judge at the New York Toy Fair with ABC Television— specifically to provide commentary on how games were evolving to improve activity levels in children.

The toy I awarded the gold medal to was the simplest. It was a pair of hard-plastic carpet skates: pieces of plastic you Velcro over your shoes that allow you to skate over carpet. I bought three pairs—two for my kids and one for me. I gave second prize to a plastic tennis racquet with a sensor in its handle; you use it to play tennis with a virtual opponent on a television screen in front of you. This was the predecessor of the Wii.

The Wii, launched at the end of 2006, was a critical moment in gaming. It demonstrated several key points. The first was that Nintendo, the manufacturer, could make a lot of money with active gaming. This is important because without a funding stream, a change in gaming will never occur. The second point was that parents lapped up the concept of active gaming. They could buy video games for their children and not feel guilty that they were condemning their children to ill health. The third point was that active gaming could be marketed as a family connector (rather than as something a child does alone). The marketing was directed at families participating in Wii together. All good. But it was the fourth point I found to be the most important.

Before the Wii became massively popular, another active game called *Dance Dance Revolution* already had a strong following. It consists of a plastic mat that is placed on the floor and is connected to the television. The mat is divided into nine numbered squares, and the television, with accompanying music, instructs users on which square to put their feet on. The songs start off slowly but get faster, and soon sweating kids are bopping around like crazy. It seemed too good to be true, a video game that made you dance.[18] Large studies examined whether deploying *Dance Dance Revolution* would help kids lose weight and become healthier.[19] To the surprise of the scientific community, it failed; there was no sustained weight loss through "exergaming," as it became known.[20] Results indicated that already active kids liked *Dance Dance Revolution*, but overweight kids could not keep up and became discouraged. After these findings were known, data on the Wii started to come out.

To play with the Wii, a user holds a thick wand that contains sensors that communicate with the console and television. To swing the virtual tennis racquet, you swing the wand. At least that is what researchers assumed. What actually happens is that kids learn to game the system. Instead of swinging their arm, they learn to simply flick their wrist. The wand senses the wrist's motion, and the racquet moves wildly on the television screen. The trouble is, a wrist flick consumes almost no calories.

I learned this the hard way when I played Wii tennis with my daughter. I was flying around the living room while she sat still, giggling and simply wriggling her wrist. Sweat poured off me; amusement emanated from her. She won the tennis match from the sofa. Data were reinforcing the early lessons I'd learned in Hong Kong.

This was the fourth point about the Wii. In games that are designed to promote activity, kids frequently learn to cheat the system; the game comes first. In another example, children had to cycle on a stationary bike to watch television, but the kids learned to bypass the lock system and watch the TV while sitting.[21]

Kids are just too smart! The game comes first. Even active gaming does not necessarily make the player more active or reverse the harm of excess sitting.

Regardless of these technical limitations, the trouble with all types of video and computer gaming is that we are overlooking that the fundamental aspects of play are broader than swinging an arm or flicking a wrist at a television screen. With recess times becoming only 20 minutes, which includes eating lunch, where will kids learn the rough-and-tumble of the playground, how to scrape their knees and interact with each other and develop a sense of social hierarchy?

I think back to the joyous yelps of the girl when she kicked a goal barefoot in the Nairobi slum and the wild happiness on the faces of the children playing in the open water faucet in the Mumbai slum. I then think of the Iowa boy killing people on his video console in the basement to ward off stress. Physical play is a vital part of happiness, and modern gamers are losing out. Modern kids are as much prisoners of cars and electronic screens as their parents—they have been sentenced to lethal sitting just as we have.

ANIMAL PLAY

On one of my trips to Nairobi, I stayed at the Stanley Hotel, an old colonial hotel frequented by the likes of author Ernest Hemingway. I was sitting in the Thorne Café with some colleagues from the Red Cross. A few tables away sat a middle-aged blond woman. "That's Jane Goodall," I was told.

The premise of Dr. Jane Goodall's work is that you cannot study chimpanzees in confined laboratories. In order to understand their true natures, you must study them in their natural ecology. I feel the same thing about human science. So much of what we discover in research labs is irrelevant because societal factors—the weather and poverty are examples—are overlooked. Jane and I began to correspond.

A few years later, Dr. Goodall wrote to me, "Have you seen our latest data?" Her most recent paper summarized the behavior of chimpanzees living in the wild as they were designed to do.[22] The report was beautiful. She demonstrated that chimpanzee play is not only critical in child development but also that play is important in adult primates.

Jane described the play of adult chimpanzees, specifically how play paralleled tool development behaviors and mental inquiry. She described how chimpanzees use shaped sticks to clear tree hollows (akin to modern gardening), how grooming is an essential part of socialization (rather like a massage) and how play-fighting is normal adult chimpanzee behavior (like "high-fiving" or back slaps). She went on to describe chimpanzee activities that resemble sports—throwing objects to each other and competitive racing. Sexual overtones and activities (including self-stimulation) were part of normal play activity too. Of course she described restfulness, napping and sitting as well, but these broke up the various types of play rather than displaced it.

Play is a forgotten part of adult human life too. Play is fun, joyous and healthy. Whether it is a spin class with friends, making out with your partner, going for a walk with a parent or playing chess on a hot day in the park—play is a pivotal part of life. Play is the pulse of creativity.

Playfulness is rare in corporate America. Adults rarely play—they email. People forsake a conversation for a text. Sometimes I too get caught up in the nonsense of modern everlasting work. How much fun have I forgone for worthless meetings? How much play have I lost for another unfunded grant application? How many games of tag have I missed with my kids? When was the last time you played? Play is one way to achieve happiness, and humans are neurologically wired to play and be happy.[23]

Now it is time for me to log off, get up and play.

17

DEFEAT THE CHAIRMAN

End Lethal Sitting!

IT IS 8 P.M. I AM ALONE HERE IN MY LONG, NARROW LABO-
ratory in Rochester, Minnesota, waiting for a mouse measurement to finish.

The lab has five white standing-height benches. Bench 1 is
filled with neatly lined-up insulin infusers for experiments in
diabetes. Bench 2 is cluttered with a precision drill, a milling
machine and dozens of pieces of electronic-development equipment; circuit boards have wires sticking out of them. Bench 3 has
kids' video gaming equipment and an array of active toys; some
are dismantled so that they can be adapted. Bench 4 is filled with
DNA analysis equipment. The last bench is Gabe and Samantha's center of operations, where our chair-release programs are
designed and tested. The place is a mess with reverse-engineered
treadmills, pieces of prefabricated standing desks and boxes of
MEMS (micro electro-mechanical systems) movement sensors.
The lab also has two annexes; one is Shelly's office, and the other
is where the NEAT (nonexercise activity thermogenesis) of the
mouse is being measured.

At the far end of the long lab, hung on hooks, are a dozen sets of magic underwear, and stacked against the wall is a pile of redundant equipment including a four-foot-long fish tank with bright blue gravel. I bought the tank at a garage sale for $25. Three years ago, 34 years after I started, I decided to try and solve why pond snails have different types of movement. When I was 11 years old, I had traced onto parchment paper that Joanne, the first pond snail I loved, moved in a sawtooth pattern. In contrast, Maurice, another snail, moved smoothly across the glass. And so, I bought the fish tank and some snails and began to record their movements using time-lapse photography.

The results were the same as what I had found in my boyhood; some snails have a jagged way of moving whereas others move smoothly. By pure chance, in 2011 I was invited to Montclair State University in New Jersey and during my lecture mentioned my early snail experiments. Afterward, a senior professor came up to me. "You're right," he said, "snails do move differently because the snail foot behaves differently from snail to snail." He explained that remarkable studies had been conducted at Stanford University where other snail-o-philes had photographed snail foot patterns 15 times per second, measured forces across their feet and used laser-illuminated gel sheets to analyze the snails' movements.[1] The researchers discovered that the snail foot not only contracts longwise, in intricately orchestrated waves, but also from side to side. The research, involving multiple species of gastropods, demonstrated that every snail has an intricate and unique way of moving. Yes! Joanne was truly different from Maurice; individuality is etched into the most primal DNA. It is just the same with people; every person has a unique way of moving—by design.

I have worked across the globe. I have watched kids playing in low-income slums, on rural Native American reservations and in inner cities. I have met students in Kenya, India, Jamaica, China and across Europe and the United States. Young people intuitively understand the need of the human body to move. They get it! Movement isn't just critical for health and intellectual vitality but for happiness. Everyone moves differently; everyone has their own style of movement, but it is universal that moving people smile. We are designed to move—people in motion are happy. Motion is the notion.

Sedentary living has swept through modern America, Europe, Japan and now China and India. The death toll runs to millions. In corporations—dozens of them—I find people sentenced to their chairs. After a day's work, employees leave work chairs to travel in car chairs to spend their leisure time in armchairs and on sofas. Go into any chair-based corporation, and you will sense the malaise. Ask any corporate board, and they will reel off the curse of growing healthcare costs and the need to bolster productivity and creative ingenuity.

The chair-based life we lead—at work, at school, in our cars and at home—has left us weakened in body, mind and spirit. Our bodies are diseased, our minds have slowed and our spirit is waning. Seated people are weak and unproductive. As a nation of chair addicts, we are falling behind. But we can change: We must because if we don't, the next generation will be even worse off.

As a society, we sit at a juncture. If we stay on this course, diabetes, obesity, cardiovascular death, cancer and dementia will ravage our generation, our children's and all those that follow. If we get up now and plan an active way forward, there is hope. Chairlessness will not cost money; in fact, the opposite. At a personal, workplace and national level, a chairless revolution—a national uprising of human movement—will improve productivity and generate revue, better health, clean air and enhanced happiness.

The good news is that there are scientifically validated solutions for your company, school, community and self. Strategies, technologies, tools and plans exist that can help you get up and stay up. I offer you a promise. If you get up from your chair, you'll be better for it.

Erich Fromm, the noted psychologist, argued that "each person's virtue" is their "unique individuality," but that, at the same time, we seek a "closeness" with others.[2] Just as *your* style of movement is unique, so too will be *your* solution for *your* chair escape. However, you can't do it alone—nor can I. The Chairman has succeeded in dulling our sense of uniqueness and separating us from each other. We must rid ourselves of The Chairman together. In closing this book, I ask for your help.

If you see someone wanting to get up, encourage them.

If you see someone rise up—whether it is against ill health, a difficult relationship or a sense of suffocation—support them.

If someone needs your help, help them.

If you need help, ask.

It someone extends a helping hand to you—take it.

If someone sits back down, nudge them up again.

If you are standing and someone stands beside you, embrace.

If someone is walking behind you, invite them forward.

Get up now. Don't be afraid.

Take the hand of the person beside you.

Because, hand in hand and step by step, the world will heal.

ACKNOWLEDGMENTS

THANK YOU TO ELISABETH DYSSEGAARD, WHO GAVE ME the liberty and support to write a book that needed writing. Natanya Wheeler kept the fire roaring—thank you.

* * *

I acknowledge the National Institutes of Health and the Mayo Foundation for funding my laboratory for the last 25 years. I stand on the shoulders of giants—too many to name. My debt of gratitude to you all cannot be quantified. Thank you to Obesity Solutions at Mayo Clinic and Arizona State University.

To the scientists who have come through my lab and with whom I have had the honor of working, I am so proud and grateful. I hope that I have done justice to your work in the pages above.

To my lab—Shelly McCrady-Spitzer, Gabriel Koepp, Chinmay Manohar and Samantha Calvin—may you all receive blessings too many to quantify, for my thanks are inadequate.

To my family and friends: You have sacrificed the most but waver the least.

NOTES

INTRODUCTION

1. Levine JA. Health-chair reform: your chair: comfortable but deadly. *Diabetes* 2010;59:2715-6.
2. Levine JA, Weisell R, Chevassus S, Martinez CD, Burlingame B, Coward WA. The work burden of women. *Science* 2001;294:812. See also Levine JA, McCrady SK, Boyne S, Smith J, Cargill K, Forrester T. Non-exercise physical activity in agricultural and urban people. *Urban Studies* 2011;48:2417-27.

CHAPTER 1: IN THE BEGINNING

1. Huang C, Xiong C, Kornfeld K. Measurements of age-related changes of physiological processes that predict lifespan of Caenorhabditis elegans. *Proceedings of the National Academy of Sciences of the United States of America.* 2004;101:8084-9.
2. Rose HE, Mayer J. Activity, calorie intake, fat storage, and the energy balance of infants. *Pediatrics* 1968;41:18-29.
3. Eriksson B, Henriksson H, Lof M, Hannestad U, Forsum E. Body-composition development during early childhood and energy expenditure in response to physical activity in 1.5-y-old children. *American Journal of Clinical Nutrition* 2012;96:567-73. Abitbol MM. Effect of posture and locomotion on energy expenditure. *American Journal of Physical Anthropology* 1988;77:191-9.
4. Haley S, Beachy J, Ivaska KK, Slater H, Smith S, Moyer-Mileur LJ. Tactile/kinesthetic stimulation (TKS) increases tibial speed of sound and urinary osteocalcin (U-MidOC and unOC) in premature infants (29–32 weeks PMA). *Bone* 2012;51:661-6.
5. Ekelund U, Yngve A, Brage S, Westerterp K, Sjostrom M. Body movement and physical activity energy expenditure in children and adolescents: how to adjust for differences in body size and age. *American Journal of Clinical Nutrition* 2004;79:851-6.

6. Lanningham-Foster LM, Jensen TB, McCrady SK, Nysse LJ, Foster RC, Levine JA. Laboratory measurement of posture allocation and physical activity in children. *Medicine and Science in Sports and Exercise* 2005;37:1800–5. Harris AM, Lanningham-Foster LM, McCrady SK, Levine JA. Nonexercise movement in elderly compared with young people. *American Journal of Physiology—Endocrinology and Metabolism* 2007;292:E1207–12. Levine JA, Lanningham-Foster LM, McCrady SK, et al. Interindividual variation in posture allocation: possible role in human obesity. *Science* 2005;307:584–6.

7. Berciano J, Infante J, Garcia A, et al. Stiff man-like syndrome and generalized myokymia in spinocerebellar ataxia type 3. *Movement Disorders: Official Journal of the Movement Disorder Society* 2006;21:1031–5. Greene PE, Dauer W. Stiff child syndrome with mutation of DYT1 gene. *Neurology* 2006;66:1456; author reply.

8. Zhong S, Israel S, Xue H, Ebstein RP, Chew SH. Monoamine oxidase A gene (MAOA) associated with attitude towards longshot risks. *PLOS One* 2009;4:e8516.

9. Macmurray J, Comings DE, Napolioni V. The gene-immune-behavioral pathway: Gamma-interferon (IFN-gamma) simultaneously coordinates susceptibility to infectious disease and harm avoidance behaviors. *Brain, Behavior, and Immunity* 2013;35:169-75. Cuypers K, De Ridder K, Kvaloy K, et al. Leisure time activities in adolescence in the presence of susceptibility genes for obesity: risk or resilience against overweight in adulthood? The HUNT study. *BMC Public Health* 2012;12:820.

10. Lordkipanidze D, Ponce de Leon MS, Margvelashvili A, et al. A complete skull from Dmanisi, Georgia, and the evolutionary biology of early Homo. *Science* (New York, NY) 2013;342:326–31.

11. Vigne JD, Briois F, Zazzo A, et al. First wave of cultivators spread to Cyprus at least 10,600 y ago. *Proceedings of the National Academy of Sciences of the United States of America* 2012;109:8445–9.

12. Dehaene S, Changeux JP. Reward-dependent learning in neuronal networks for planning and decision making. *Progress in Brain Research* 2000;126:217–29. Borday C, Wrobel L, Fortin G, Champagnat J, Thaeron-Antono C, Thoby-Brisson M. Developmental gene control of brainstem function: views from the embryo. *Progress in Biophysics and Molecular Biology* 2004;84:89–106.

13. Lordkipanidze D, Ponce de Leon MS, Margvelashvili A, et al. A complete skull from Dmanisi, Georgia, and the evolutionary biology of early Homo. *Science* 2013;342:326–31. Kawamichi H, Kikuchi Y, Noriuchi M, Senoo A, Ueno S. Distinct neural correlates underlying two- and three-dimensional mental rotations using three-dimensional objects. *Brain Research* 2007;1144:117–26.

14. Sirotkina I. When did "scientific psychology" begin in Russia? *Physis; Rivista Internazionale di Storia Della Scienza* 2006;43:239–71.

15. Imbert M, Buisseret P. Receptive field characteristics and plastic properties of visual cortical cells in kittens reared with or without visual experience. Experimental Brain Research/Experimentelle Hirnforschung Experimentation Cerebrale 1975;22:25–36. Vital-Durand F, Jeannerod M. Eye movement related activity in the visual cortex of dark-reared kittens. *Electroencephalography and Clinical Neurophysiology* 1975;38:295–301.

16. Mora F. Successful brain aging: plasticity, environmental enrichment, and lifestyle. Dialogues in Clinical Neuroscience 2013;15:45–52. Rosa AM, Silva MF, Ferreira S, Murta J, Castelo-Branco M. Plasticity in the human visual cortex: an ophthalmology-based perspective. *BioMed Research International* 2013;568354:1-13.

17. Keys A, Anderson JT, Brozek J. Weight gain from simple overeating. I. Character of the tissue gained. *Metabolism* 1955;4:427–32. Grande F, Anderson JT, Keys A. Changes of basal metabolic rate in man in semistarvation and refeeding. *Journal of Applied Physiology* 1958;12:230–8. Keys A, Brozek J, Henschel A, Mickelson O, Taylor HL. *The Biology of Human Starvation*. Minneapolis: University of Minnesota Press; 1950.

18. Hebebrand J, Exner C, Hebebrand K, et al. Hyperactivity in patients with anorexia nervosa and in semistarved rats: evidence for a pivotal role of hypoleptinemia. *Physiology & Behavior* 2003;79:25–37. Novak CM, Jiang X, Wang C, Teske JA, Kotz CM, Levine JA. Caloric restriction and physical activity in zebrafish (Danio rerio). *Neuroscience Letters* 2005;383:99–104. Scrimshaw NS. The phenomenon of famine. *Annual Review of Nutrition* 1987;7:1–21. Merkt JR, Taylor CR. "Metabolic switch" for desert survival. *Proceedings of the National Academy of Sciences USA* 1994;91:12313–6.

19. Levine JA. Health-chair reform: your chair: comfortable but deadly. Diabetes 2010;59:2715-6.

CHAPTER 2: FEED ME, MOVE ME

1. Lavoisier, A. *Methode de nomenclature chimique.* Paris: The Academy of Sciences, France; 1747.

2. Benedict FG. An apparatus for studying the respiratory exchange. *American Journal of Physiology* 1909;24:345–74.

3. Hamilton MT, Hamilton DG, Zderic TW. Exercise physiology versus inactivity physiology: an essential concept for understanding lipoprotein lipase regulation. *Exercise and Sport Sciences Review* 2004;32:161–6.

4. Black AE, Coward WA, Cole TJ, Prentice AM. Human energy expenditure in affluent societies: an analysis of 574 doubly-labelled water measurements. *European Journal of Clinical Nutrition* 1996;50:72-92.

5. Levine JA, Schleusner SJ, Jensen MD. Energy expenditure of non-exercise activity. *American Journal of Clinical Nutrition* 2000;72: 1451–4.

6. Levine JA, Schleusner SJ, Jensen MD. Energy expenditure of nonexercise activity. *American Journal of Clinical Nutrition* 2000;72:1451–4.

7. Lanningham-Foster L, Nysse LJ, Levine JA. Labor saved, calories lost: the energetic impact of domestic labor-saving devices. *Obesity Research* 2003;11:1178–81.

8. James WP. The epidemiology of obesity: the size of the problem. *Journal of Internal Medicine* 2008;263:336–52.

9. Wang YC, Colditz GA, Kuntz KM. Forecasting the obesity epidemic in the aging U.S. population. *Obesity* (Silver Spring) 2007;15:2855–65.

10. Sikorski C, Riedel C, Luppa M, et al. Perception of overweight and obesity from different angles: a qualitative study. *Scandinavian Journal of Public Health* May 2012;40(3):271–7. O'Brien KS, Latner JD, Ebneter D, Hunter JA. Obesity discrimination: the role of physical appearance, personal ideology, and anti-fat prejudice. *International Journal of Obesity* (Lond). 2013 Mar;37(3):455-60.

11. Cawley J, Meyerhoefer C. The medical care costs of obesity: an instrumental variables approach. *Journal of Health Economics* 2012;31(1):219–30.

12. Levine JA. Nonexercise activity thermogenesis (NEAT): environment and biology. *American Journal of Physiology—Endocrinology and Metabolism* 2004;286:E675–85. Levine JA. Nonexercise activity thermogenesis—liberating the life-force. *Journal of Internal Medicine* 2007;262:273–87. Levine JA, Eberhardt NL, Jensen MD. Role of nonexercise activity thermogenesis in resistance to fat gain in humans. *Science* 1999;283:212–4.

13. Jones, JM. In U.S., More Would Like to Lose Weight Than Are Trying To. *Gallup*. November 20, 2009. http://www.gallup.com/poll/124448/in-u.s.-more-lose-weight-than-trying-to.aspx.

14. Levine JA, Lanningham-Foster LM, McCrady SK, et al. Interindividual variation in posture allocation: possible role in human obesity. *Science* 2005;307:584–6. Levine J, Melanson EL, Westerterp KR, Hill JO. Measurement of the components of nonexercise activity thermogenesis. *American Journal of Physiology—Endocrinology and Metabolism* 2001;281:E670–5.

15. Morgane PJ, Stern WC. *Rhythms of the Biogenic Amines in the Brain and Sleep.* Tokyo: Igaku Shoin; 1974.

CHAPTER 3: THE BRAIN STRAIN

1. Kiwaki K, Kotz CM, Wang C, Lanningham-Foster L, Levine JA. Orexin A (hypocretin 1) injected into hypothalamic paraventricular

nucleus and spontaneous physical activity in rats. *American Journal of Physiology—Endocrinology and Metabolism* 2003;2:2.

2. Novak CM, Escande C, Burghardt PR, et al. Spontaneous activity, economy of activity, and resistance to diet-induced obesity in rats bred for high intrinsic aerobic capacity. *Hormone and Behavior* 2010;58(3):355–67. Ecker RD, Goerss SJ, Meyer FB, Cohen-Gadol AA, Britton JW, Levine JA. Vision of the future: initial experience with intraoperative real-time high-resolution dynamic infrared imaging. Technical note. *Journal of Neurosurgery* 2002;97:1460–71.

3. Sabbahi MA, Fox AM, Druffle C. Do joint receptors modulate the motoneuron excitability? *Electromyography and Clinical Neurophysiology* 1990;30:387–96.

4. Mora F. Successful brain aging: plasticity, environmental enrichment, and lifestyle. *Dialogues in Clinical Neuroscience* 2013;15:45–52. Rosa AM, Silva MF, Ferreira S, Murta J, Castelo-Branco M. Plasticity in the Human visual cortex: an ophthalmology-based perspective. *Bio-Medical Research International* 2013;2013:1-13. Dixon KJ, Hilber W, Speare S, Willson ML, Bower AJ, Sherrard RM. Post-lesion transcommissural olivocerebellar reinnervation improves motor function following unilateral pedunculotomy in the neonatal rat. *Experimental Neurology* 2005;196:254–65. Pysh JJ, Weiss GM. Exercise during development induces an increase in Purkinje cell dendritic tree size. *Science* 1979;206:230–2.

CHAPTER 4: DESPITE YOUR CHAIR, YOU ARE AN INDIVIDUAL

1. Levine JA. Obesity in China: causes and solutions. *Chinese Medical Journal* (Engl) 2008;121:1043–50.

2. Dr. Edward Smith. On the nourishment of the distressed operatives. Appendix V. P320-456. Public Health. Fifth Report of The Medical Officer of the Privy Council. The House of Commons, London 1862.

3. Delisle H, Ntandou-Bouzitou G, Agueh V, Sodjinou R, Fayomi B. Urbanisation, nutrition transition and cardiometabolic risk: the Benin study. *The British Journal of Nutrition* 2012;107:1534-44. Ding D, Sallis JF, Hovell MF, et al. Physical activity and sedentary behaviours among rural adults in Suixi, China: a cross-sectional study. *The International Journal of Behavioral Nutrition and Physical Activity* 2011;8:37.4. Weng X, Liu Y, Ma J, Wang W, Yang G, Caballero B. An urban-rural comparison of the prevalence of the metabolic syndrome in Eastern China. *Public Health Nutrition* 2007;10:131-6. Levine JA, McCrady SK, Boyne S, Smith J, Cargill K, Forrester T. Non-exercise physical activity in agricultural and urban people. *Urban Studies* (Edinburgh, Scotland) 2011;48:2417-27.

CHAPTER 5: THE CHAIR-CURSED BODY

1. Diet and exercise in noninsulin-dependent diabetes mellitus. *National Institutes of Health Consensus Development Conference Statement* 1986 Dec 8-10;6(8):1-21. Levine JA. Health-chair reform: your chair: comfortable but deadly. *Diabetes* 2010;59:2715-6.

2. Statistics About Diabetes. American Diabetes Association. http://www.diabetes.org/diabetes-basics/statistics/?loc=db-slabnav. Accessed August 1, 2011.

3. Manohar C, Levine JA, Nandy DK, et al. The effect of walking on postprandial glycemic excursion in patients with type 1 diabetes and healthy people. *Diabetes Care* 2012;35:2493-9.

4. Dunstan DW, Barr EL, Healy GN, et al. Television viewing time and mortality: the Australian Diabetes, Obesity and Lifestyle Study (AusDiab). *Circulation* 2010;121:384-91.

5. Duncan GE. Exercise, fitness, and cardiovascular disease risk in type 2 diabetes and the metabolic syndrome. *Current Diabetes Reports* 2006;6:29-35. Vuori IM. Health benefits of physical activity with special reference to interaction with diet. *Public Health Nutrition* 2001;4:517-28. Kujala UM, Kaprio J, Koskenvuo M. Diabetes in a population-based series of twin pairs discordant for leisure sedentariness. *Diabetologia* 2000;43:259. Pi-Sunyer FX. Comorbidities of overweight and obesity: current evidence and research issues. *Medicine and Science in Sports and Exercise* 1999;31:S602-8. Connelly PW, Petrasovits A, Stachenko S, MacLean DR, Little JA, Chockalingam A. Prevalence of high plasma triglyceride combined with low HDL-C levels and its association with smoking, hypertension, obesity, diabetes, sedentariness and LDL-C levels in the Canadian population. Canadian Heart Health Surveys Research Group. *Canadian Journal of Cardiology* 1999;15:428-33. de Souza Santos Machado V, Valadares AL, da Costa-Paiva LS, Moraes SS, Pinto-Neto AM. Multimorbidity and associated factors in Brazilian women aged 40 to 65 years: a population-based study. *Menopause* (New York, NY) 2012;19:569-75. Adeniyi AF, Fasanmade AA, Aiyegbusi OS, Uloko AE. Physical activity levels of type 2 diabetes patients seen at the outpatient diabetes clinics of two tertiary health institutions in Nigeria. *Nigerian Quarterly Journal of Hospital Medicine* 2010;20:165-70. Koepp GA, Manohar CU, McCrady-Spitzer SK, Levine JA. Scalable office-based health care. *Health Services Management Research* 2011;24:69-74. Orozco Beltran D, de la Sen Fernandez C, Guillen VG, Munuera CC, Perez JN. Diabetes mellitus and cardiovascular risk. Is integrated therapy of type 2 diabetes and cardiovascular risk factors necessary?. *Atencion Primaria/Sociedad Espanola de Medicina de Familia y Comunitaria* 2010;42 Suppl 1:16-23. Duteil D, Chambon C, Ali F, et al.

The transcriptional coregulators TIF2 and SRC-1 regulate energy homeostasis by modulating mitochondrial respiration in skeletal muscles. *Cell Metabolism* 2010;12:496–508. de Leon AC, Rodriguez JC, Coello SD, et al. Lifestyle and treatment adherence of type 2 diabetes mellitus people in the Canary Islands. *Revista Espanola de Salud Publica* 2009;83:567–75. Carolino ID, Molena-Fernandes CA, Tasca RS, Marcon SS, Cuman RK. Risk factors in patients with type 2 diabetes mellitus. *Revista Latino-Americana de Enfermagem* 2008;16:238–44. Capon AG. The way we live in our cities. *Medical Journal of Australia* 2007;187:658–61.

6. Zderic TW, Hamilton MT. Physical inactivity amplifies the sensitivity of skeletal muscle to the lipid-induced downregulation of lipoprotein lipase activity. *Journal of Applied Physiology* 2006;100:249–57. Hamilton MT, Hamilton DG, Zderic TW. Role of low energy expenditure and sitting in obesity, metabolic syndrome, type 2 diabetes, and cardiovascular disease. *Diabetes* 2007;56:2655–67. Dunstan DW, Kingwell BA, Larsen R, et al. Breaking up prolonged sitting reduces postprandial glucose and insulin responses. *Diabetes Care* 2012;35:976–83.

7. Bey L, Hamilton MT. Suppression of skeletal muscle lipoprotein lipase activity during physical inactivity: a molecular reason to maintain daily low-intensity activity. *The Journal of Physiology* 2003;551:673-82.

8. Koba S, Tanaka H, Maruyama C, et al. Physical activity in the Japan population: association with blood lipid levels and effects in reducing cardiovascular and all-cause mortality. *Journal of Atherosclerosis and Thrombosis* 2011;18:833–45.

9. Ekblom-Bak E, Hellenius ML, Ekblom O, Engstrom LM, Ekblom B. Independent associations of physical activity and cardiovascular fitness with cardiovascular risk in adults. *European Journal of Cardiovascular Prevention and Rehabilitation: Official Journal of the European Society of Cardiology, Working Groups on Epidemiology & Prevention and Cardiac Rehabilitation and Exercise Physiology* 2010;17:175–80.

10. van de Laar RJ, Stehouwer CD, Prins MH, van Mechelen W, Twisk JW, Ferreira I. Self-reported time spent watching television is associated with arterial stiffness in young adults: the Amsterdam Growth and Health Longitudinal Study. *British Journal of Sports Medicine* 2014;48:256-64.

11. Rietsch K, Eccard JA, Scheffler C. Decreased external skeletal robustness due to reduced physical activity? *American Journal of Human Biology: The Official Journal of the Human Biology Council* 2013;25:404–10.

12. Van der Ploeg HP, Chey T, Korda RJ, Banks E, Bauman A. Sitting time and all-cause mortality risk in 222,497 Australian adults. *Archives of Internal Medicine* 2012;172:494-500.

13. National Cancer Institute Factsheet: Physical Activity and Cancer. http://www.cancer.gov/cancertopics/factsheet/prevention/physical activity.

14. Hildebrand JS, Gapstur SM, Campbell PT, Gaudet MM, Patel AV. Recreational physical activity and leisure-time sitting in relation to postmenopausal breast cancer risk. *Cancer Epidemiology, Biomarkers & Prevention* 2013;22:1906-12.

15. Sitting for long periods "is bad for your health." BBC News Health. October 14, 2012. http://www.bbc.co.uk/news/health-19910888.

16. Hamilton MT, Healy GN, Dunstan DW, Zderic TW, Owen N. Too little exercise and too much sitting: inactivity physiology and the need for new recommendations on sedentary behavior. *Current Cardiovascular Risk Reports* 2008;2:292-8.

17. Dunlop D, Song J, Arnston E, et al. Sedentary Time in U.S. Older Adults Associated With Disability in Activities of Daily Living Independent of Physical Activity. *Journal of Physical Activity & Health* 2014, http://dx.doi.org/10.1123/jpah.2013-0311.

18. Sitting less for adults. HeartFoundation.org. http://www.heartfoundation.org.au/SiteCollectionDocuments/HW-PA-SittingLess-Adults.pdf; Reducing sedentary behaviors: Sitting less and standing more. American College of Sports Medicine. http://www.acsm.org/docs/brochures/reducing-sedentary-behaviors-sitting-less-and-moving-more.pdf; Canadian Sedentary Behaviour Guidelines for Children and Youth. *Applied Physiology, Nutrition, and Metabolism* 2011;36(1):59-64, 10.1139/H11-012. http://www.nrcresearchpress.com/doi/abs/10.1139/H11-012#.Uvma2aVurnc.

CHAPTER 6: THE CHAIR-CURSED MIND

1. Yancey AK, Wold CM, McCarthy WJ, et al. Physical inactivity and overweight among Los Angeles County adults. *American Journal of Preventive Medicine* 2004;27:146–52. Vance DE, Wadley VG, Ball KK, Roenker DL, Rizzo M. The effects of physical activity and sedentary behavior on cognitive health in older adults. *Journal of Aging and Physical Activity* 2005;13:294–313. Paluska SA, Schwenk TL. Physical activity and mental health: current concepts. *Sports Medicine* 2000;29:167–80.

2. Sacco P, Thickbroom GW, Byrnes ML, Mastaglia FL. Changes in corticomotor excitability after fatiguing muscle contractions. *Muscle & Nerve* 2000;23:1840–6. Dunn AL, Trivedi MH, O'Neal HA. Physical activity dose-response effects on outcomes of depression and anxiety. *Medicine and Science in Sports and Exercise* 2001;33:S587–97; discussion 609–10. Stenzel-Poore MP, Heinrichs SC, Rivest S, Koob GF, Vale WW. Overproduction of corticotropin-releasing factor in

transgenic mice: a genetic model of anxiogenic behavior. *Journal of Neuroscience* 1994;14:2579–84.

3. Byron K, Khazanchi S, Nazarian D. The relationship between stressors and creativity: a meta-analysis examining competing theoretical models. *Journal of Applied Psychology* 2010;95:201–12.

4. Klem ML, Wing RR, McGuire MT, Seagle HM, Hill JO. Psychological symptoms in individuals successful at long-term maintenance of weight loss. *Health Psychology* 1998;17:336–45. DePue JD, Clark MM, Ruggiero L, Medeiros ML, Pera V, Jr. Maintenance of weight loss: a needs assessment. *Obesity Research* 1995;3:241–8. Cachelin FM, Striegel-Moore RH, Brownell KD. Beliefs about weight gain and attitudes toward relapse in a sample of women and men with obesity. *Obesity Research* 1998;6:231–7.

5. Byron K, Khazanchi S, Nazarian D. The relationship between stressors and creativity: a meta-analysis examining competing theoretical models. *Journal of Applied Psychology* 2010;95:201–12.

6. Byron K, Khazanchi S, Nazarian D. The relationship between stressors and creativity: a meta-analysis examining competing theoretical models. *Journal of Applied Psychology* 2010;95:201–12. Biondi M, Picardi A. Psychological stress and neuroendocrine function in humans: the last two decades of research. *Psychotherapy and Psychosomatics* 1999;68:114–50. Belkic K, Nedic O. Workplace stressors and lifestyle-related cancer risk factors among female physicians: assessment using the Occupational Stress Index. *Journal of Occupational Health* 2007;49:61–71.

7. Sims EA, Bray GA, Danforth E, Jr., et al. Experimental obesity in man. VI. The effect of variations in intake of carbohydrate on carbohydrate, lipid, and cortisol metabolism. *Hormone and Metabolic Research* 1974;Suppl 4:70–7.

8. Siervo M, Wells JC, Cizza G. The contribution of psychosocial stress to the obesity epidemic: an evolutionary approach. *Hormone and Metabolic Research* 2009;41:261–70. Gantz I, Fong TM. The melanocortin system. *Am J Physiol Endocrinol Metab* 2003;284:E468-74.

9. Vozarova B, Weyer C, Snitker S, et al. Effect of cortisol on muscle sympathetic nerve activity in Pima Indians and Caucasians. *Journal of Clinical Endocrinology and Metabolism* 2003;88:3218–26.

10. McMahon BT, West SL, Mansouri M, Belongia L. Workplace discrimination and diabetes: the EEOC Americans with Disabilities Act research project. *Work* 2005;25:9–18. Giel KE, Thiel A, Teufel M, Mayer J, Zipfel S. Weight bias in work settings—a qualitative review. *Obesity Facts* 2010;3:33–40.

11. Calvin AD, Carter RE, Adachi T, et al. Effects of experimental sleep restriction on caloric intake and activity energy expenditure. *Chest* 2013;144:79–86.

12. Rasch B, Born J. About sleep's role in memory. *Physiological Reviews* 2013;93:681-766.
13. Milner CE, Cote KA. Benefits of napping in healthy adults: impact of nap length, time of day, age, and experience with napping. *Journal of Sleep Research* 2009;18:272–81.

CHAPTER 7: THE CHAIR-CURSED CAR

1. Huston HR, Anglin D, Eckstein M. Drive-by shootings by violent street gangs in Los Angeles: a five-year review from 1989 to 1993. *Academic Emergency Medicine: Official Journal of the Society for Academic Emergency Medicine* 1996;3:300–3. Robinson PL, Boscardin WJ, George SM, Teklehaimanot S, Heslin KC, Bluthenthal RN. The effect of urban street gang densities on small area homicide incidence in a large metropolitan county, 1994-2002. *Journal of Urban Health: Bulletin of the New York Academy of Medicine* 2009;86:511–23.
2. Gorzelany, J. The world's most traffic-congested cities. *Forbes,* April 25, 2013. http://www.forbes.com/sites/jimgorzelany/2013/04/25/the-worlds-most-traffic-congested-cities/.
3. Schrank D, Eisele B, Lomax T. TTI's 2012 Urban Mobility Report. December 2012. http://d2dtl5nnlpfr0r.cloudfront.net/tti.tamu.edu/documents/mobility-report-2012.pdf.
4. Maizlish N, Woodcock J, Co S, Ostro B, Fanai A, Fairley D. Health cobenefits and transportation-related reductions in greenhouse gas emissions in the San Francisco Bay area. *American Journal of Public Health* 2013;103:703–9.
5. PricewaterhouseCoopers. The 150 richest cities in the world by GDP in 2005. March 11, 2007. http://www.citymayors.com/statistics/richest-cities-2005.html.
6. Xia T, Zhang Y, Crabb S, Shah P. Cobenefits of replacing car trips with alternative transportation: a review of evidence and methodological issues. *Journal of Environmental and Public Health* 2013;2013:797312:1–14.
7. Xia T, Zhang Y, Crabb S, Shah P. Cobenefits of replacing car trips with alternative transportation: a review of evidence and methodological issues. *Journal of Environmental and Public Health* 2013;2013:797312:1–14.
8. Xia T, Zhang Y, Crabb S, Shah P. Cobenefits of replacing car trips with alternative transportation: a review of evidence and methodological issues. *Journal of Environmental and Public Health* 2013;2013:797312:1–14.
9. Woodcock J, Givoni M, Morgan AS. Health impact modelling of active travel visions for England and Wales using an Integrated

Transport and Health Impact Modelling Tool (ITHIM). *PLOS One* 2013;8:e51462.

10. Maizlish N, Woodcock J, Co S, Ostro B, Fanai A, Fairley D. Health cobenefits and transportation-related reductions in greenhouse gas emissions in the San Francisco Bay area. *American Journal of Public Health* 2013;103:703–9.

11. Owen N, Bauman A, Brown W. Too much sitting: a novel and important predictor of chronic disease risk? *British Journal of Sports Medicine* 2009;43:81–3.

CHAPTER 8: THE CHAIRMAN'S VISION

1. Melzer-Lange MD. Violence and associated high-risk health behavior in adolescents. Substance abuse, sexually transmitted diseases, and pregnancy of adolescents. *Pediatric Clinics of North America* 1998;45:307–17.

2. Katsnelson A. Polypill improves adherence but fails to win all scientists' hearts. *Nature Medicine* 2013;19:1192. Gaziano JM. Progress with the polypill? *JAMA: The Journal of the American Medical Association* 2013;310:910–1.

3. Light J. The education industry: the corporate takeover of public schools. *CorpWatch*, July 8, 1998. http://corpwatch.org/article.php ?id=889.

4. Webb S. One in ten modern couples live separately because they feel "emotionally safer" if they keep their independence. *Daily Mail* April 23, 2013. http://www.dailymail.co.uk/news/article-2313414/How -growing-number-modern-couples-living-apart-feel-emotionally -safe-keeping-independence.html–ixzz2kI9Knyhx.

CHAPTER 9: SOLUTIONS

1. Infographic: Sitting so much should scare you. JustStand.org. http:// www.juststand.org/tabid/800/language/en-US/default.aspx.

2. Levine JA, Lanningham-Foster LM, McCrady SK, et al. Interindividual variation in posture allocation: possible role in human obesity. *Science* 2005;307:584–6. McCrady SK, Levine JA. Sedentariness at work: how much do we really sit? *Obesity* (Silver Spring) 2009;17:2103–5. Levine JA, McCrady SK, Boyne S, Smith J, Cargill K, Forrester T. Non-exercise physical activity in agricultural and urban people. *Urban Studies* (Edinburgh, Scotland) 2011;48:2417–27.

3. Cash TF. Body-image attitudes: evaluation, investment, and affect. *Perception and Motor Skills* 1994;78:1168–70. Frith CD, Frith U. Mechanisms of social cognition. *Annual Review of Psychology* 2011;63:287–313.

4. Kozuki Y, Kennedy MG. Cultural incommensurability in psychodynamic psychotherapy in Western and Japanese traditions. *Journal of Nursing Scholarship: An Official Publication of Sigma Theta Tau International Honor Society of Nursing/Sigma Theta Tau* 2004;36:30–8.

CHAPTER 10: INVENT!

1. Bouten CV, Verboeket-van de Venne WP, Westerterp KR, Verduin M, Janssen JD. Daily physical activity assessment: comparison between movement registration and doubly labeled water. *Journal of Applied Physiology* 1996;81:1019–26.

2. Societies Directory, Cambridge Footlights. http://www.cusu.cam .ac.uk/societies/directory/footlights/.

3. Foster RC, Lanningham-Foster LM, Manohar C, et al. Precision and accuracy of an ankle-worn accelerometer-based pedometer in step counting and energy expenditure. *Preventive Medicine* 2005;41:778–83. Manohar C, McCrady S, Pavlidis IT, Levine JA. An accelerometer-based earpiece to monitor and quantify physical activity. *Journal of Physical Activity & Health* 2009;6:781–9. Manohar CU, McCrady SK, Fujiki Y, Pavlidis IT, Levine JA. Evaluation of the accuracy of a triaxial accelerometer embedded into a cell phone platform for measuring physical activity. *Journal of Obesity and Weight Loss Therapy* 2011;1:3309-14. Manohar CU, Koepp GA, McCrady-Spitzer SK, Levine JA. A stand-alone accelerometer system for free-living individuals to measure and promote physical activity. *Infant, Child, & Adolescent Nutrition* 2012;4:222–9. Manohar CU, McCrady SK, Fujiki Y, Pavlidis IT, Levine JA. Evaluation of the accuracy of a triaxial accelerometer embedded into a cell phone platform for measuring physical activity. *Journal of Obesity and Weight Loss Therapy* 2011;1:3309-14.

4. Bouten CV, Verboeket-van de Venne WP, Westerterp KR, Verduin M, Janssen JD. Daily physical activity assessment: comparison between movement registration and doubly labeled water. *Journal of Applied Physiology* 1996;81:1019–26. Westerterp KR, Bouten CV. Physical activity assessment: comparison between movement registration and doubly labeled water method. *Zeitschrift für Ernährungswissenschaft* 1997;36:263–7. Bouten CV, Koekkoek KT, Verduin M, Kodde R, Janssen JD. A triaxial accelerometer and portable data processing unit for the assessment of daily physical activity. *IEEE Transactions on Biomedical Engineering* 1997;44:136–47. Bouten CV, Sauren AA, Verduin M, Janssen JD. Effects of placement and orientation of body-fixed accelerometers on the assessment of energy expenditure during walking. *Medical & Biological Engineering & Computing* 1997;35:50–6. Westerterp KR, Verboeket-van

de Venne WP, Bouten CV, de Graaf C, van het Hof KH, Weststrate JA. Energy expenditure and physical activity in subjects consuming full-or reduced-fat products as part of their normal diet. *British Journal of Nutrition* 1996;76:785–95. Bouten CV, van Marken Lichtenbelt WD, Westerterp KR. Body mass index and daily physical activity in anorexia nervosa. *Medicine and Science in Sports and Exercise* 1996;28:967–73. Pannemans DL, Bouten CV, Westerterp KR. 24 h energy expenditure during a standardized activity protocol in young and elderly men. *European Journal of Clinical Nutrition* 1995;49:49–56. Bouten CV, Westerterp KR, Verduin M, Janssen JD. Assessment of energy expenditure for physical activity using a triaxial accelerometer. *Medicine and Science in Sports and Exercise* 1994;26:1516–23. Bouten CVC. Asssessment of daily physical activity by registration of body movement. PhD thesis, Einhoven University of Technology 1995.

5. Manohar CU, McCrady SK, Fujiki Y, Pavlidis IT, Levine JA. Evaluation of the accuracy of a triaxial accelerometer embedded into a cell phone platform for measuring physical activity. *Journal of Obesity and Weight Loss Therapy* 2011;1:3309-14.

6. McCrady-Spitzer SK, Levine JA. Integrated electronic platforms for weight loss. *Expert Review of Medical Devices* 2010;7:201–7.

7. McCrady-Spitzer SK, Levine JA. Integrated electronic platforms for weight loss. *Expert Review of Medical Devices* 2010;7:201–7.

CHAPTER 11: WORK!

1. Church TS, Thomas DM, Tudor-Locke C, et al. Trends over 5 decades in U.S. occupation-related physical activity and their associations with obesity. *PLOS One* 2011;6:e19657.

2. Infographic. Sitting so much should scare you. JustStand.org. http://www.juststand.org/tabid/800/language/en-US/default.aspx.

3. Ng SW, Popkin BM. Time use and physical activity: a shift away from movement across the globe. *Obesity reviews: an official journal of the International Association for the Study of Obesity* 2012;13:659–80.

4. Bauman A, Ainsworth BE, Sallis JF, et al. The descriptive epidemiology of sitting. A 20-country comparison using the International Physical Activity Questionnaire (IPAQ). *American Journal of Preventive Medicine* 2011;41:228–35.

5. The Facts About Diabetes: A Leading Cause of Death in the U.S. National Diabetes Education Program. http://ndep.nih.gov/diabetes-facts/.

6. Centers for Disease Control and Prevention. Vital signs: prevalence, treatment, and control of hypertension—United States, 1999-2002 and 2005-2008. *Morbidity and Mortality Weekly Report* 2011;60(4):103-8.

7. Levine JA, Koepp GA. Federal health-care reform: opportunities for obesity prevention. *Obesity* (Silver Spring);19:897–9.

8. Chronic diseases: The power to prevent, the call to control: At a glance 2009. Centers for Disease Control and Prevention. http://www.cdc.gov/chronicdisease/resources/publications/aag/chronic.htm.

9. LaDou J, Rohm T. The international electronics industry. *International Journal of Occupational and Environmental Health* 1998;4:1–18. Kawakami N. Improvement of work environment. Sangyo eiseigaku zasshi. *Journal of Occupational Health* 2002;44:95–9. Tudor-Locke C, Leonardi C, Johnson WD, Katzmarzyk PT. Time spent in physical activity and sedentary behaviors on the working day: the American time use survey. *Journal of Occupational and Environmental Medicine/American College of Occupational and Environmental Medicine* 2011;53:1382–7.

10. Wakefield MA, Loken B, Hornik RC. Use of mass media campaigns to change health behaviour. *Lancet* 2010;376:1261-71.

11. Grady D. New weight-loss focus: the lean and the restless. *New York Times.* May 24, 2005. http://www.nytimes.com/2005/05/24/health/nutrition/24wigg.html?pagewanted=all&_r=0.

12. Walking while you work. ABCNews, October 5, 2007. http://abcnews.go.com/GMA/WaterCooler/story?id=3771802.

13. Levine JA, Weisell R, Chevassus S, Martinez CD, Burlingame B, Coward WA. The work burden of women. *Science* 2001;294:812.

14. Soares MJ, Shetty PS. Basal metabolic rates and metabolic economy in chronic undernutrition. *European Journal of Clinical Nutrition* 1991;45:363–73. Shetty PS. Adaptive changes in basal metabolic rate and lean body mass in chronic undernutrition. *Human Nutrition—Clinical Nutrition* 1984;38:443–51. James WP, Shetty PS. Metabolic adaptation and energy requirements in developing countries. *Human Nutrition—Clinical Nutrition* 1982;36:331–6.

15. Levine JA, Weisell R, Chevassus S, Martinez CD, Burlingame B. Looking at child labor. *Science* 2002;296:1025–6.

16. Morris JN, Hardman AE. Walking to health. *Sports Medicine* 1997;23:306–32. Mann JI. Can dietary intervention produce long-term reduction in insulin resistance? *British Journal of Nutrition* 2000;83 Suppl 1:S169–72. Tremblay A. Physical activity and obesity. *Best Practice & Research Clinical Endocrinology & Metabolism* 1999;13:121–9.

17. McGorry P. Prevention, innovation and implementation science in mental health: the next wave of reform. *British Journal of Psychiatry Supplement* 2013;54:s3–4. Fitzgerald CJ, Danner KM. Evolution in the office: how evolutionary psychology can increase employee health, happiness, and productivity. *Evolutionary Psychology: An International Journal of Evolutionary Approaches to Psychology and*

Behavior 2012;10:770–81. Kerfoot KM. The pursuit of happiness, science, and effective staffing: the leader's challenge. *Nursing Economics* 2012;30:305–6. Zydiak GP. 7 tips to increase your professional happiness productivity. *Medical Economics* 2010;87:41–2, 7. Fritz C, Yankelevich M, Zarubin A, Barger P. Happy, healthy, and productive: the role of detachment from work during nonwork time. *Journal of Applied Psychology* 2010;95:977–83.

18. Lovett RA. Sitting all day at work can be dangerous for your health. *StarTribune*. July 28, 2013. http://m.startribune.com/lifestyle/?id=21 7156181.

19. Koepp GA, Manohar CU, McCrady-Spitzer SK, Levine JA. Scalable office-based health care. *Health Services Management Research* 2011;24:69–74. Koepp GA, Manohar CU, McCrady-Spitzer SK, et al. Treadmill desks: A one-year prospective trial. *Obesity* 2012; 21:705-11.

CHAPTER 12: LEARN!

1. National Collaborative on Child Obesity Research. Childhood Obesity in the United States. http://www.nccor.org/downloads/Child hoodObesity_020509.pdf.

2. National Collaborative on Child Obesity Research. Childhood Obesity in the United States. http://www.nccor.org/downloads/Child hoodObesity_020509.pdf.

3. Daviglus ML, Lloyd-Jones DM, Pirzada A. Preventing cardiovascular disease in the 21st century: therapeutic and preventive implications of current evidence. *American Journal of Cardiovascular Drugs* 2006;6:87–101. Rosenthal T, Gavras I. Fixed-drug combinations as first-line treatment for hypertension. *Progress in Cardiovascular Disease* 2006;48:416–25. Jamieson MJ, Naghavi M. Multi-constituent cardiovascular pills (MCCP)—challenges and promises of population-based prophylactic drug therapy for prevention of heart attack. *Current Pharmaceutical Design* 2007;13:1069–76. Athyros VG, Tziomalos K, Mikhailidis DP, et al. Do we need a statin-nicotinic acid-aspirin mini-polypill to treat combined hyperlipidaemia? *Expert Opinion on Pharmacotherapy* 2007;8:2267–77. Franco OH, Karnik K, Bonneux L. The future of metabolic syndrome and cardiovascular disease prevention: polyhype or polyhope? Tales from the polyera. *Hormone and Metabolic Research* 2007;39:627–31.

4. Daviglus ML, Lloyd-Jones DM, Pirzada A. Preventing cardiovascular disease in the 21st century: therapeutic and preventive implications of current evidence. *American Journal of Cardiovascular Drugs* 2006;6:87–101.

5. Levine JA. Obesity in China: causes and solutions. *Chinese Medical Journal* 2008;121:1043–50.

6. Wu Y, Lau BD, Bleich S, et al. Future Research Needs for Child-hood Obesity Prevention Programs: Identification of Future Research Needs From Comparative Effectiveness Review No. 115. Rockville MD2013.

7. Erskine HE, Ferrari AJ, Nelson P, et al. Research review: epidemio-logical modelling of attention-deficit/hyperactivity disorder and con-duct disorder for the Global Burden of Disease Study 2010. *Journal of Child Psychology and Psychiatry* 2013;54:1263-74.

8. Lanningham-Foster L, Foster RC, McCrady SK, et al. Changing the school environment to increase physical activity in children. *Obesity* (Silver Spring) 2008;16:1849-53.

9. Koepp GA, Snedden BJ, Flynn L, Puccinelli D, Huntsman B, Levine JA. Feasibility Analysis of Standing Desks for Sixth Graders. *Infant, Child, & Adolescent Nutrition* 2012;4:89-92.

10. National collaborative on child obesity research. childhood obesity in the united states. http://www.nccor.org/downloads/Childhood Obesity_020509.pdf.

CHAPTER 13: GET UP!, STEP 1: GET PERSONAL!

1. *Military psychology; a Soviet view.* Shelyag VV, Glotochkin AD, Pla-tonov KK, eds. Moscow: Military Publishing House of the Ministry of Defense CCCP, 1972.

2. Bouchard TJ, Jr., McGue M. Familial studies of intelligence: a review. *Science* 1981;212:1055–9. Bohman M, Cloninger CR, Sigvardsson S, von Knorring AL. Predisposition to petty criminality in Swed-ish adoptees. I. Genetic and environmental heterogeneity. *Archives of General Psychiatry* 1982;39:1233–41. Davies G, Tenesa A, Pay-ton A, et al. Genome-wide association studies establish that human intelligence is highly heritable and polygenic. *Molecular Psychiatry* 2011;16:996–1005.

3. Mutch DM, Clement K. Genetics of human obesity. *Best Practice & Research Clinical Endocrinology & Metabolism* 2006;20:647-64.

4. Lyubomirsky S, Ross L. Changes in attractiveness of elected, rejected, and precluded alternatives: a comparison of happy and unhappy indi-viduals. *Journal of Personality and Social Psychology* 1999;76:988-1007

5. Bregman P. How (and why) to stop multitasking. 2010. http://blogs .hbr.org/2010/05/how-and-why-to-stop-multitaski/.

CHAPTER 14: GET UP!, STEP 2: PLAN!

1. Barnes PM, Adams PF, Powell-Griner E. Health characteristics of the American Indian or Alaska Native adult population: United States, 2004-2008. *National Health Statistics Reports* 2010:1-22.

2. Locke D. Clean living, throwing punches, and the secret to long life. *Ojibwe Inaajimowin: The Story As It's Told.* October 2013;15(10):4-5. http://millelacsband.com/wp-content/uploads/2013/12/inaa_octo ber2013.pdf.

3. Singh J, Prentice AM, Diaz E, et al. Energy expenditure of Gambian women during peak agricultural activity measured by the doubly-labelled water method. *British Journal of Nutrition* 1989;62:315–29.

CHAPTER 15: GET UP!, STEP 3: WEAPONS!

1. Gallagher P, Yancy WS, Jr., Jeffreys AS, et al. Patient self-efficacy and spouse perception of spousal support are associated with lower patient weight: baseline results from a spousal support behavioral intervention. *Psychology, Health & Medicine* 2013;18:175-81.

2. Gullickson G. Man of the Year. *Echo,* December 19, 2013. http://www.echomag.com/archives/features/633/year-in-review/man-of -the-year.php.

CHAPTER 16: GET UP!, STEP 4: PLAY!

1. Fedewa AL, Ahn S. The effects of physical activity and physical fitness on children's achievement and cognitive outcomes: a meta-analysis. *Research Quarterly for Exercise & Sport* 2011;82:521–35. Fox KR. Childhood obesity and the role of physical activity. *Journal of the Royal Society of Health* 2004;124:34–9. Saelens BE, Epstein LH. Behavioral engineering of activity choice in obese children. *International Journal of Obesity and Related Metabolic Disorders* 1998;22:275–7.

2. Mellecker RR, McManus AM, Lanningham-Foster LM, Levine JA. The feasibility of ambulatory screen time in children. *International Journal of Pediatric Obesity* 2009;4:106–11. Mellecker RR, Lanningham-Foster L, Levine JA, McManus AM. Energy intake during activity enhanced video game play. *Appetite* 2010;55:343–7. Moore LC, Harris CV, Bradlyn AS. Exploring the relationship between parental concern and the management of childhood obesity. *Maternal and Child Health Journal* 2012;16:902-8 Khan LK, Sobush K, Keener D, et al. Recommended community strategies and measurements to prevent obesity in the United States. *MMWR Recommendations and Reports* 2009;58:1–26.

3. Kuss DJ. Internet gaming addiction: current perspectives. *Psychology Research And Behavior Management* 2013;6:125-37.

4. DFC Intelligence. Consumer trends in virtual goods and download-able games in North America and Europe. March 26, 2010. http://www.dfcint.com/wp/?p=272.

5. *Internet Gaming Disorder* May 2013. http://www.dsm5.org/Docu ments/Internet%20Gaming%20Disorder%20Fact%20Sheet.pdf.

6. Karmali L. World of Warcraft Down to 7.7 million subscribers. IGN .com. July 26, 2013. http://www.ign.com/articles/2013/07/26/world -of-warcraft-down-to-77-million-subscribers.

7. Petry NM, O'Brien CP. Internet gaming disorder and the DSM-5. *Addiction* (Abingdon, England) 2013;108:1186-7.

8. Lanningham-Foster L, Foster RC, McCrady SK, Jensen TB, Mitre N, Levine JA. Activity-promoting video games and increased energy expenditure. *Journal of Pediatrics* 2009;154:819-23. Mitre N, Foster RC, Lanningham-Foster L, Levine JA. The energy expenditure of an activity-promoting video game compared to sedentary video games and TV watching. *Journal of Pediatric Endocrinology and Metabolism* 2011;24:689-95.

9. Kuss DJ. Internet gaming addiction: current perspectives. *Psychology Research And Behavior Management* 2013;6:125-37.

10. Kuss DJ. Internet gaming addiction: current perspectives. *Psychology Research And Behavior Management* 2013;6:125-37.

11. Levine JA. Poverty and obesity in the U.S. Diabetes 2011;60:2667-8. Levine JA. Health-chair reform: your chair: comfortable but deadly. *Diabetes* 2010;59:2715-6.

12. Kawamichi H, Kikuchi Y, Noriuchi M, Senoo A, Ueno S. Distinct neural correlates underlying two- and three-dimensional mental rotations using three-dimensional objects. *Brain Research* 2007;1144:117-26. Moriyama M, Ohno-Matsui K, Modegi T, et al. Quantitative analyses of high-resolution 3D MR images of highly myopic eyes to determine their shapes. *Investigative Ophthalmology & Visual Science* 2012;53:4510-8. Romero MC, Van Dromme I, Janssen P. Responses to two-dimensional shapes in the macaque anterior intraparietal area. *European Journal of Neuroscience* 2012;36:2324-34. Mysore SG, Vogels R, Raiguel SE, Todd JT, Orban GA. The selectivity of neurons in the macaque fundus of the superior temporal area for three-dimensional structure from motion. *Journal of Neuroscience: The Official Journal of the Society for Neuroscience* 2010;30:15491—508. Preston TJ, Kourtzi Z, Welchman AE. Adaptive estimation of three-dimensional structure in the human brain. *Journal of Neuroscience: The Official Journal of the Society for Neuroscience* 2009;29:1688-98. Creem-Regehr SH, Lee JN. Neural representations of graspable objects: are tools special? *Cognitive Brain Research* 2005;22:457-69.

13. Baukol PV, RA; Levine, JA. Community specific daily activity in Northern Plains American Indian Youth. *Fourth World Journal* 2012;11:95-104.

14. Harris KM, Gordon-Larsen P, Chantala K, Udry JR. Longitudinal trends in race/ethnic disparities in leading health indicators from adolescence to young adulthood. *Archives of Pediatric and Adolescent Medicine* 2006;160:74–81. Saylors K, Daliparthy N. Violence against Native women in substance abuse treatment. *American Indian and Alaska Native Mental Health Research* 2006;13:32–51. Yuan NP, Koss MP, Polacca M, Goldman D. Risk factors for physical assault and rape among six Native American tribes. *Journal of Interpersonal Violence* 2006;21:1566–90.

15. Bearinger LH, Pettingell S, Resnick MD, Skay CL, Potthoff SJ, Eichhorn J. Violence perpetration among urban American Indian youth: can protection offset risk? *Archives of Pediatrics & Adolescent Medicine* 2005;159:270-7. Rutman S, Park A, Castor M, Taualii M, Forquera R. Urban American Indian and Alaska Native youth: youth risk behavior survey 1997-2003. *Maternal and Child Health Journal* 2008;12 Suppl 1:76-81.

16. Lanningham-Foster L, Foster RC, McCrady SK, Jensen TB, Mitre N, Levine JA. Activity-promoting video games and increased energy expenditure. *Journal of Pediatrics* 2009;154:819–23. Mitre N, Foster RC, Lanningham-Foster L, Levine JA. The energy expenditure of an activity-promoting video game compared to sedentary video games and TV watching. *Journal of Pediatric Endocrinology and Metabolism* 2011;24:689–95. Lanningham-Foster L, Jensen TB, Foster RC, et al. Energy expenditure of sedentary screen time compared with active screen time for children. *Pediatrics* 2006;118:e1831–5.

17. Mellecker RR, McManus AM, Lanningham-Foster LM, Levine JA. The feasibility of ambulatory screen time in children. *International Journal of Pediatric Obesity* 2009;4:106–11. Mellecker RR, Lanningham-Foster L, Levine JA, McManus AM. Energy intake during activity enhanced video game play. *Appetite* 2010;55:343–7.

18. Lanningham-Foster L, Foster RC, McCrady SK, Jensen TB, Mitre N, Levine JA. Activity-promoting video games and increased energy expenditure. *Journal of Pediatrics* 2009;154:819–23.

19. Berkey CS, Rockett HR, Gillman MW, Colditz GA. One-year changes in activity and in inactivity among 10- to 15-year-old boys and girls: relationship to change in body mass index. *Pediatrics* 2003;111:836–43. Christison A, Khan HA. Exergaming for health: a community-based pediatric weight management program using active video gaming. *Clinical Pediatrics* 2012;51:382–8. Radon K, Furbeck B, Thomas S, Siegfried W, Nowak D, von Kries R. Feasibility of activity-promoting video games among obese adolescents and young adults in a clinical setting. *Journal of Science and Medicine in Sport/ Sports Medicine Australia* 2011;14:42–5.

20. Lamboglia CM, da Silva VT, de Vasconcelos Filho JE, et al. Exergaming as a strategic tool in the fight against childhood obesity: a systematic review. *Journal of Obesity* 2013;2013:1-8.
21. Faith MS, Berman N, Heo M, et al. Effects of contingent television on physical activity and television viewing in obese children. *Pediatrics* 2001;107:1043–8.
22. Whiten A, Goodall J, McGrew WC, et al. Cultures in chimpanzees. *Nature* 1999;399:682–5.
23. Blum K, Oscar-Berman M, Bowirrat A, et al. Neuropsychiatric Genetics of Happiness, Friendships, and Politics: Hypothesizing Homophily ("Birds of a Feather Flock Together") as a Function of Reward Gene Polymorphisms. *Journal Of Genetic Syndrome & Gene Therapy* 2012;3:1-17.

CHAPTER 17: DEFEAT THE CHAIRMAN

1. Lai JH, del Alamo JC, Rodriguez-Rodriguez J, Lasheras JC. The mechanics of the adhesive locomotion of terrestrial gastropods. *The Journal of Experimental Biology* 2010;213:3920-33.
2. Fromm E. *Man for himself. Inquiry into the psychology of ethics.* New York: Rinehart and Company. 1947.

INDEX